Positive Options for Sjögren's Syndrome

Ordering

Trade bookstores in the U.S. and Canada please contact:

Publishers Group West
1700 Fourth Street, Berkeley CA 94710
Phone: (800) 788-3123   Fax: (800) 351-5073

Hunter House books are available at bulk discounts for textbook course adoptions; to qualifying community, health-care, and government organizations; and for special promotions and fund-raising.
For details please contact:

Special Sales Department
Hunter House Inc., PO Box 2914, Alameda CA 94501-0914
Phone: (510) 865-5282   Fax: (510) 865-4295
E-mail: ordering@hunterhouse.com

Individuals can order our books from most bookstores, by calling
(800) 266-5592, or from our website at **www.hunterhouse.com**

Project Credits

Cover Design: Brian Dittmar Graphic Design
Book Production: Hunter House
Copy Editor: Holly Knight
Proofreader: John David Marion
Indexer: Nancy D. Peterson
Acquisitions Editor: Jeanne Brondino
Editor: Alexandra Mummery
Publishing Assistant: Herman Leung
Publishing Intern: Shelley McGuire
Publicist: Jillian Steinberger
Foreign Rights Coordinator: Elisabeth Wohofsky
Customer Service Manager: Christina Sverdrup
Order Fulfillment: Joe Winebarger, Washul Lakdhon
Administrator: Theresa Nelson
Computer Support: Peter Eichelberger
Publisher: Kiran S. Rana

Positive Options

for

Sjögren's Syndrome

Self-Help and Treatment

Sue Dyson

Hunter House Inc., Publishers
PO Box 2914
Alameda CA 94501-0914

Library of Congress Cataloging-in-Publication Data

Dyson, Sue.
Positive options for Sjögren's syndrome : self-help and treatment / Sue
Dyson.-- 1st American ed.
p. cm. -- (Positive options for health series)
"First published as Living with Sjögren's Syndrome in Great Britain in 2005
by Sheldon Press."
Summary: "Provides clear explanations and practical information for
sufferers of Sjögren's syndrome, the most common rheumatic-type
autoimmune disease. Presents and evaluates a full range of treatment
options, conventional and alternative, providing assessments of their
possible benefits and side-effects"--Provided by publisher.
Includes index.
ISBN-13: 978-0-89793-473-2 (pbk.)
ISBN-10: 0-89793-473-3 (pbk.)
1. Sjögren's syndrome--Popular works. 2. Sjögren's syndrome--Treatment--
Popular works. 3. Sjögren, Henrik, 1899-1986. I. Dyson, Sue. Living with
Sjögren's syndrome. II. Title. III. Series.
RC647.5.S5D97 2005
616.7'75--dc22   2005013712

Manufactured in the United States of America

9 8 7 6 5 4 3 2   First Edition   10 11 12 13 14

Contents

Foreword

Chronic diseases are wearing and debilitating. This is more so when existing medical and surgical treatments can offer only limited benefits. In this situation sufferers have to search for coping strategies that work for them. What works today may not work tomorrow. Imagination, tenacity, and flexibility are essential. Sjögren's syndrome, named after Swedish opthalmologist Dr. Henrick Sjögren, certainly fits into the above description. Oddly, this condition may cause additional frustration and irritation for sufferers in that they often look well but feel awful.

What Dr. Sjögren recognized was the association of dry eyes and mouth, sometimes in association with arthritis in a predominantly female group of patients. The other key observation was that the affected glands did not have the hallmarks of chronic infection, even though they were inflamed. Some twenty years later the concept of alterations in the body's immune system—so called autoimmunity—began to emerge. What Dr. Sjögren described seventy years ago can now be categorized into various types and subtypes. This exercise is not simply an academic nicety, because the differing forms have varying clinical and laboratory abnormalities and run differing courses.

Making the diagnosis can be a somewhat protracted exercise. Although Sjögren's syndrome is not rare, probably affecting about 1 percent of the population, it is not a diagnosis that leaps into people's minds. It has not received extensive coverage in the media and, because the symptoms may be vague and nonspecific in the early stages, people are often given alternative explanations, such as anxiety or depression.

Certain features of the disease, in particular the dryness of the eyes and mouth, are common to all types of Sjögren's, but other features are very much tailor made to the individual affected. Even within the common strands of dry eyes and mouth, some sufferers find topical lubricants and gels helpful, whereas others require more aggressive therapies. However, it is fair to say that many of the dramatic medical advances, which have radically altered the outlook for many autoimmune diseases, have been singularly disappointing for Sjögren's syndrome and, worse still, are often associated with unacceptable side effects.

In this book, Sue Dyson takes us through the features of the disease and how it expresses itself, using her experiences and those of others as illustrations. She also thoroughly explores the various conventional and alternative treatments that are available. Individuals affected by this disease will probably find this menu approach very helpful. Some may or may not be relevant to you, others may not work, but some probably will.

This text provides a balanced introduction to those recently diagnosed and will allow them to frame questions for their healthcare professionals. For patients with established disease, the range of therapies and strategies described may take them onto fruitful avenues not previously explored. Just reading how others have coped with chronic disorders may be supportive and enlightening to everyone with this syndrome.

This is a book I can thoroughly recommend. It complements other patient information literature that is available and explores in great detail many of the issues that are not covered in often busy and hurried consultations with doctors, dentists, and opticians. As Sue stresses, remaining positive is critical. Chronic illnesses are a bit like gardens: Either you are on top of them, or they are on top of you. Rarely is there a comfortable neutral position.

Dr. Ian Griffiths

Consultant rheumatologist at the Freeman Hospital
Newcastle-upon-Tyne, United Kingdom

Acknowledgments

The author and publisher would like to thank Ian Griffiths, consultant rheumatologist at the Freeman Hospital, Newcastle-upon-Tyne, for checking and correcting this book.

Important Note

The material in this book is intended to provide a review of information regarding Sjögren's syndrome. Every effort has been made to provide accurate and dependable information. The contents of this book have been compiled through professional research and in consultation with medical professionals. However, health-care professionals have differing opinions, and advances in medical and scientific research are made very quickly, so some of the information may become outdated.

Therefore, the publisher, authors, and editors, as well as the professionals quoted in the book, cannot be held responsible for any error, omission, or dated material. The authors and publisher assume no responsibility for any outcome of applying the information in this book in a program of self-care or under the care of a licensed practitioner. If you have questions concerning your health, or about the application of the information described in this book, consult a qualified health-care professional.

Introduction

Sjögren's syndrome is a somewhat mysterious entity—not much is known about it, and it is equally hard to pronounce! If you have just been diagnosed with Sjögren's syndrome, the chances are you had never even heard of it before your doctor gave you a diagnosis. And yet it is estimated that there are 4 million people with Sjögren's syndrome in the United States.

With the ever-increasing awareness of autoimmune diseases, however, recognition of Sjögren's syndrome is growing, and some doctors believe that it is more common than initially thought. In addition to its hallmark symptoms of dry eyes and dry mouth, Sjögren's also causes a range of other symptoms that can lead to it being confused with other chronic conditions. For example, aching joints and deep fatigue, two common symptoms, may lead to an initial diagnosis of arthritis, a common misdiagnosis. It is common to be referred to a rheumatologist for arthritis, and then given a diagnosis of Sjögren's later on. This path mirrors the identification of Sjögren's as a syndrome, which arose from a study of patients with arthritis. Some people may also have Sjögren's in combination with another autoimmune disease, such as lupus.

Sjögren's is capable of affecting just about any part of the body, including the organs, so it is helpful to be aware of the potential complications of Sjögren's. In my own case, for example, it has caused nerve damage to my face (leading to a lopsided smile) and may very well have contributed to my bowel and bladder problems. As my rheumatologist once said: You can blame almost anything on Sjögren's syndrome. At the same time, it is important to seek the opinion of a doctor about any new symptoms that arise rather than attributing them to Sjögren's without investigation.

The good news is that, for most people, Sjögren's manifests itself in a relatively benign form. Some people may never experience
anything more than slightly dry eyes and mouth, which can easily
be treated with eye drops, artificial saliva, and plenty of fluids.
Others may go through days of fatigue but otherwise lead a full life.
It is a question of learning about your individual pattern of Sjögren's and trying treatments and adapting your lifestyle accord-
ingly.

On the whole, there are a great deal of things you can do to
help yourself, and that is what this book is about. Taking control of
your life can help keep you positive and inventive about ways of
coping with a long-term condition like Sjögren's. We'll be looking
at such areas as your feelings, alternative therapies, relaxation, exercise, nutrition, socializing, pregnancy, family life—all the topics
you probably won't get a chance to discuss with your doctor but
that must be considered if you're going to get the best out of life.

This book will also look at the various diagnostic and therapeutic aspects of medical treatment that you can expect to en-
counter along the way. Perhaps you have just been diagnosed and
may now be wondering exactly how your life will be affected. With
the help of this book, I hope you will discover that diagnosis isn't
the end of the story and that it really is amazing what you can do if
you put your mind to it.

Chapter 1

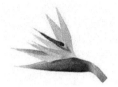

What Is Sjögren's Syndrome?

Jean

Much of the time I feel fine, if a bit less energetic than I used to be. When my Sjögren's is active, I feel vaguely fluey and really tired and I'll often need to take a few hours of complete rest before my energy comes back. My mouth feels hot and dry and I usually drink lots of ice water. My eyes are very sensitive to light, especially sunlight, and I have to wear sunglasses in all sorts of embarrassing places, such as subway stations, church, and concerts! I also have very dry skin and tend to get rashes.

So what is Sjögren's syndrome (pronounced 'Sher-gren' or 'Show-gren')? With its hallmark symptoms of dry eyes and a dry mouth, that are often accompanied by fatigue and generalized aching, this condition has only been recognized relatively recently and certainly isn't yet a household word.

A syndrome is a group of related symptoms or signs that occur together to characterize a particular condition. Sjögren's syndrome (sometimes called SJS for short) was described by the Polish doctor Johann Mikulicz-Radecki in 1898 and was at first called Mikulicz syndrome. However, this name was later applied to other conditions that cause dryness and is therefore no longer used specifically to describe this disease, and so the name of the syndrome was changed to Sjögren's syndrome (SJS) to acknowledge the work of Dr. Henrik Sjögren, a Swedish ophthalmologist who also described the set of symptoms specific to Sjögren's.

In 1933 he noticed that there was a connection in his patients between severely dry eyes, dry mouth, and arthritis. Later on, it was recognized that patients could have the dry eyes and mouth without the arthritis. Sjögren described this syndrome in his doctoral thesis.

There are two kinds of Sjögren's syndrome that have been defined:

1. *Primary Sjögren's syndrome* occurs on its own with no other associated disease.

2. *Secondary Sjögren's syndrome* is associated with another autoimmune disease, like rheumatoid arthritis, lupus, or primary biliary cirrhosis.

Sjögren's Syndrome and the Immune System

The fact that Sjögren's is an autoimmune disease may raise fears that you have a weak immune system and are therefore more prone to disease, but with Sjögren's it appears that the immune system is, in fact, overactive.

Almost fifty years ago Sjögren's was defined as a "chronic autoimmune rheumatic disease characterized by the sicca complex (decreased tears and saliva), resulting in keratoconjunctivitis sicca (dry eyes) and xerostomia (dry mouth)." Of course, as many Sjögren's patients know all too well, the symptoms can be much more wide ranging than that and the illness can attack just about any part of the body. It is very common for patients to suffer from fatigue and aching joints, for example, as well as dry airways and skin, and the disorder can cause problems as diverse as numbness, skin rashes, and an underactive thyroid gland. Inflammation is a common problem, and it can affect the joints, muscles, nerves, kidneys, thyroid gland, and indeed just about any area of the body.

In a Sjögren's patient, the body's immune system gets mixed up and starts attacking the body's own healthy cells as if they were invaders, such as germs. Since the body attacks itself, this type of condition is called an autoimmune syndrome, and although this mix-up happens in all autoimmune diseases, in Sjögren's, the body's primary target is the body's moisture-producing glands. The white cells, or lymphocytes, attack and invade the glands, and this gradually reduces the glands' ability to produce fluids—tears and saliva—hence the dry eyes and mouth that are the primary symptoms of Sjögren's.

During this autoimmune process, the immune system produces antibodies, exactly as if the body was fighting off a virus. These are called autoantibodies, and since their presence can be detected through blood tests, testing for them can help doctors to diagnose whether or not a patient is suffering from Sjögren's.

Sjögren's is not by any means the only autoimmune disease. There are a whole host of them. Some, like lupus and Sjögren's, may affect many organs of the body; while others, like thyroid disease or pernicious anemia, may single out just one organ. All are related in some way and sometimes display similar symptoms, which can complicate the doctor's job of diagnosis. You may find that you are, or have been, tested for some of the following:

- Lupus (systemic lupus erythematosus, or SLE)

- Scleroderma

- Rheumatoid arthritis

- Polymyositis

- Dermatomyositis

- Thyroid disease

- Autoimmune liver disease

Patients with secondary Sjögren's syndrome will also suffer from some other kind of autoimmune disorder, like the ones listed on the previous page. Two of the most common include rheumatoid arthritis and lupus.

Rheumatoid Arthritis

Rheumatoid arthritis (RA) is a very common autoimmune disease affecting approximately one in one hundred people, in which the body attacks itself, leading to inflammation and damage to the joints. Because the illness is systemic (it affects the whole body), other organs can also be affected, and additional symptoms include fatigue and depression.

As with Sjögren's, more women than men are affected. For every man who suffers from this disorder, three women get it. Women also tend to develop it sooner and more severely—it typically first manifests itself in women who are in their thirties and in men who are in their forties.

Some of the symptoms of rheumatoid arthritis are the same as those that occur in other forms of arthritis and some are quite distinct. As with other autoimmune diseases, experts believe it originates with part of the body's defense system, which attacks the body's own tissue, mistaking it for foreign invaders, such as bacteria or viruses. There are more than one hundred types of arthritis, not all of which involve inflammation or inflammation alone. Nevertheless, arthritis tends to involve common symptoms, including warmth, pain, soreness, tenderness, or irritation accompanied by swelling and redness in one or more joints; stiffness in the joint, especially on waking or after inactivity; and difficulty or pain in moving the joint that results in loss of movement and flexibility. Treatments consist of management (rest, pain management, lifestyle changes, and sometimes diet), drugs, and, in severe cases, surgery. Research into RA is ongoing, and areas of investigation include genetic inheritance and gene therapy, the role of hormones (given that so many more women than men contract the disease), the nature of the immune system, and new drugs designed to halt the inflammation process.

Lupus

Lupus is an autoimmune disease in which a person's immune system becomes overactive and attacks the body, causing damage and dysfunction. Lupus is called a multisystem disease because it can reach many different parts of the body, sometimes affecting major body organs.

Some patients with lupus have a very mild condition, which can be treated with simple medications, whereas others can have serious, life-threatening complications. Like Sjögren's, lupus is more common in women—in fact, 90 percent of sufferers are women—and tends to occur in those between the ages of fifteen and forty. The reason for this is unknown, as is the cause, though certain factors, such as direct sunlight, can make the condition worse. As with Sjögren's, appearances can be deceptive—the typical "butterfly"-shaped rash on the face gives a false impression of glowing good health, while the unfortunate sufferer may be feeling far from healthy.

Symptoms include extreme fatigue, joint pain, muscle aches, anemia, and general malaise, and lupus may mimic other diseases, such as multiple sclerosis and rheumatoid arthritis, making it difficult to diagnose. It is believed to affect more than 1.5 million people in the United States. Options for lupus sufferers have improved in recent years, with the development of better drug treatments and greater awareness of the condition.

Fibromyalgia (FM)—Another Related Condition

Fibromyalgia (FM), formerly sometimes called fibrositis, is not well understood and is characterized by a group of symptoms involving pain and fatigue. Some estimate that as many as half of all people with Sjögren's also suffer from FM. As with Sjögren's and lupus,

FM can be a frustrating condition in that people often don't look ill, but they feel awful. Other symptoms include poor or unrefreshing sleep, depression, forgetfulness, poor circulation, headaches including migraine, an urgent need to pass water, and irritable bowel–type symptoms. Sometimes people with FM experience the same kind of debilitating fatigue as those with Sjögren's—an exhaustion that may come on suddenly and necessitate the sufferer putting her feet up for absolute rest.

The pain affects the muscles and ligaments, but not usually the joints, and is often described as a burning kind of pain. Doctors tend to diagnose it by applying pressure to several tender points around the body. In a person with normal health, such pressure may be uncomfortable but not painful; in someone with FM, it may cause considerable discomfort or pain.

The cause of FM isn't known, although some research has linked the condition with sleep deprivation. It is also thought that a trigger may be needed for FM to develop, such as a virus or any incident that traumatizes the body, like childbirth or a car accident. Treatment includes drugs to control the pain and improve sleep, though lifestyle modifications can be very effective in helping people manage their condition. These include rest, diet, exercise, stress management, and warmth or heat to make the body more comfortable.

Symptoms

Dry mouth and dry eyes are the two key symptoms of Sjögren's syndrome. The absence of salivation and tearing—two seemingly insignificant functions that are largely taken for granted—can have a significant effect on the health of the mouth and the eyes.

Dry Mouth

Julia

On bad days, my mouth sometimes feels as if it's full of cotton, and I find it more difficult than usual to swallow and taste. Certain foods make my tongue sore, such as tomato ketchup, vinegar, pineapple, oranges, and apples. My sense of smell has changed, and I have developed a dry cough. I also get occasional mouth infections.

In Sjögren's, the body's immune system gradually attacks and destroys the saliva glands, which are located in the mouth and cheeks and underneath the chin. Most of them are tiny (especially the ones on the inside of your lip), and people don't tend to be aware of them until they stop working properly.

Drinking more liquids helps, but sometimes even doing that isn't enough to replace the natural moisture in the mouth because the body is producing diminishing amounts of saliva. Imagine eating ten crackers in succession without a drink! As the dryness worsens, eating and swallowing become progressively more difficult. Some people may also find that they develop a dry cough or have difficulty in speaking, and it is quite common to undergo changes in smell and taste.

Saliva is more than just water. It contains important substances that are designed to help protect the teeth from decay. Consequently, when not enough saliva is present, the result tends to be more cavities and more scolding from the dentist! Indeed, it is often the dentist who spots the first tell-tale signs and recommends the patient to be tested for Sjögren's.

Along with dryness and dental decay comes soreness. A dry mouth easily becomes damaged, cracked, and inflamed. Mucous membranes can feel as if they are burning. Infections can get into the gums, and thrush may become a constant problem. In severe cases, the parotid glands on either side of the face (the ones that swell up when someone has the mumps) can puff up and become inflamed or infected.

Another complication can be a sore throat and problems with hoarseness in the voice, which can be serious if you have a job like singing or teaching, where you need a good, strong, clear voice. Fortunately, you can help protect your voice, and the measures you can take are discussed in Chapter 3.

Dry Eyes

Mark

At first I kept running to the mirror to see if I had an eyelash stuck in my left eye, in particular, but there was never anything there. I feel as though there's a bit of sand all the time in my eyes—on a windy day it's as though specks of grit are constantly being blown into my eyes. They feel hot and very sensitive.

Feeling like you have a bit of grit in your eye but being unable to see it is one of the classic signs of Sjögren's. As the immune system attacks the lachrymal glands (the ones that produce tears), the glands produce less and less of the liquid that is vital for lubricating the eyeball. Doctors call this *aqueous tear deficiency*, because the amount of water in the tears is reduced. Lack of moisture makes the eyes more sensitive to both chemical and physical environmental irritants, producing the gritty sensation. Without tears, the eye's delicate surface is vulnerable to damage every time the eyelid flicks over it or if a speck of dirt gets in. There may also be an abnormal sensitivity to light, and/or little trails of mucus on the cornea, and the white of the eye may become red. In severe cases, infection and corneal erosions may occur.

Needless to say, a dry eye is also extremely uncomfortable, so most people will seek medical help and advice a long time before any serious damage has been done. I, for example, used to wear soft, disposable contact lenses occasionally for acting or singing on stage. Gradually I became aware of the fact that they just weren't comfortable any more. They felt gritty, and when I took them out, my eyes felt sore. A visit to the optician confirmed that I was not producing enough tears, and I was prescribed eye-drops that replace the moisture.

Is the Dryness Really Due to Sjögren's?

It is important to realize that a number of other conditions can mimic the pattern of the dryness of Sjögren's syndrome, particularly in the early phase. A combination of fatigue, a feeling of dryness, and widespread aching may, for example, present as part of depression, FM, or hypothyroidism.

Other diseases influence the brain centers that control tears and saliva. People with multiple sclerosis and diabetes may have dryness of the eyes and mouth, as these diseases affect the brain processes involved with the control of certain sensory and motor functions.

In addition to problems with the neural activation of the glands, other medical conditions can cause the glands to be dry or to become enlarged. People with FM may suffer fatigue, memory loss, aching muscles and, occasionally, depression. They very frequently have dryness of the eyes and mouth. These symptoms may be very disabling but, unlike in Sjögren's, the gland itself is not damaged. It is important to distinguish these symptoms from Sjögren's syndrome itself, which is an autoimmune process that does destroy the gland, because the treatments are different.

Decreased tear and salivary production also occurs as part of the normal aging process, and a variety of commonly used drugs interfere with the neurogenic stimulus to the tear and salivary glands—the so-called anticholinergic drugs. Examples of these are antidepressants, antihistamines, and some drugs used to treat Parkinson's disease.

Other Problems

Mandy

I blamed our old mattress for my discomfort and made my husband go out and buy an expensive new one—the aches and pains were just as bad! I sometimes get so tired that I fall asleep on the sofa watching TV with the kids, and a few times we've missed their after-school activities, which I feel very guilty about. I've also got dreadful teeth and have had to have one removed!

Unfortunately, both primary and secondary Sjögren's syndrome can affect other parts of the body as well, causing problems in the skin, joints, lungs, kidneys, blood vessels, and nervous system—though usually not all at once. The symptoms are all linked to the immune system's attack on the body's moisture-producing glands. In other words, the autoimmune response that causes dry eyes and mouth can cause inflammation throughout the body.

Even patients with mild primary Sjögren's commonly suffer from more than just dry eyes and mouth. For example, aching joints and extreme tiredness are very frequent problems, though not necessarily as a result of damage caused by the immune system. These additional problems are known as systemic or extra-glandular symptoms.

It's important to emphasize that you will probably not have all of these symptoms. Grouped together as follows, they do make a fearsome list; however, you are unlikely to have them all and may indeed only suffer from one or two. Sjögren's can be very idiosyncratic—part of the reason it's hard to diagnose. Other common symptoms include the following:

- *Tooth problems.* Because saliva helps protect the teeth from bacteria, you are more prone to developing cavities if your mouth is dry.

- *Vision problems.* Dry eyes can lead to light sensitivity, blurred vision, and corneal ulcers.

- *Aches and pains.* Pain in the muscles and/or joints is common, and in many cases is worsened by FM, which is thought to be a problem for 50–60 percent of Sjögren's patients. This kind of pain is also a feature of other autoimmune diseases like lupus and rheumatoid arthritis and, indeed, some people may have a diagnosis of two of these or of all three. Whether these diagnoses are correct or not is another matter. Diagnosing Sjögren's can be fraught with difficulty, and it has been suggested that some people are over-diagnosed and may, in fact, only have Sjögren's.

- *Extreme fatigue* (also a symptom of FM). Poor sleeping patterns, often due to frequent trips to the bathroom at night because of all the extra fluid drunk during the day, don't help the situation!

- *Dry skin and rashes.* About half of those with Sjögren's have dry skin. Some experience only itching (though it can be severe and can lead to infection if a person scratches vigorously), some develop rashes, and others develop cracked, split skin that is easily infected.

- *Sinusitis and sinus infections.* Paradoxically, even when someone's eyes and mouth are dry, they may suffer postnasal drip, and dehydration tends to make it worse.

- *Respiratory problems.* Some people may suffer upper airway and lung problems, such as dry cough, bronchitis, or even pneumonia.

- *Fever.* Some people find that they run a slight temperature, often described as "feeling fluey."

- *Swollen lymph nodes* (e.g., in the groin).

- *Swollen glands.* The parotid glands at the side of the face are among the glands that can become swollen in people with this condition. The swelling may be more common when you are dehydrated.

- *Impaired memory and concentration.* Mental functions can be affected by the release of inflammatory substances by the immune system.

- *Vaginal dryness.* Because Sjögren's often develops after the age of forty, some women take no action because they assume that the dryness is simply part of the menopausal or perimenopausal process. Women need to remember that it is important to investigate each symptom for its true cause so treatments can be identified.

◆ *Digestive problems.* Dry mouth can extend right down the esophagus and all the way to the stomach, pancreas, and liver. These internal organs can all become inflamed, resulting in problems like painful swallowing, heartburn and reflux, abdominal pain and swelling, loss of appetite, diarrhea, and irritable bowel syndrome.

◆ *Inflammatory problems with internal organs.* Sometimes the heart, liver and, most commonly, the kidneys can become involved.

◆ *Nerve problems.* Inflammation can sometimes attack the nerves in the arms, legs, or extremities and cause pain, numbness, and tingling in the fingers (which may be due to carpal tunnel syndrome); in the legs or arms (due to a peripheral neuropathy); or in the face or throat (cranial neuropathy).

Sjögren's Syndrome and Lymphoma?

Many people with Sjögren's worry about developing cancer of the lymph nodes, or lymphoma. The early studies into Sjögren's syndrome in the 1960s found that lymphoma occurred forty-four times more frequently in Sjögren's patients than it did in age- and sex-matched people without the syndrome. However, some of the treatments for Sjögren's that were used at that time, such as irradiation of the swollen parotid glands, may have increased the risk of lymphoma.

Subsequent studies have confirmed an increased risk of lymphoma, but have also shed more light on this worrying aspect. It turns out that only a subset of patients with Sjögren's are at increased risk, and these are the patients with particular abnormal antibodies, known as the Ro and La antibodies (see page 22). Patients with secondary Sjögren's, or those with only the dry eyes or mouth and without the abnormal antibodies, do not have an increase in lymphoma. Moreover, in those people who are unlucky enough to develop lymphoma, it is often at the very mild end of the lymphoma spectrum, sometimes known as maltoma. In fact, these lymphomas often follow such a mild course that the specialists, usually hematologists or oncologists, may well decide not to treat them, but merely keep them under observation. Overall, over a ten-year period lymphoma may develop in about 5 percent of those who have both the syndrome and the immunological abnormalities.

The most common symptom of lymphoma is a painless swelling of the lymph nodes in the neck, underarm, or groin. The salivary glands may also be swollen, usually in an asymmetrical fashion. Other symptoms may include fever, night sweats, constant fatigue, unexplained weight loss, itchy skin, and red patches on the skin. However, these can be due to a host of other factors apart from lymphoma, so do consult your doctor for advice and diagnosis. Ultimately the diagnosis rests on the results of a biopsy from the suspect site. A biopsy also allows the doctor to classify the nature of the lymphoma (if that is what is found) and plan appropriate treatment.

Who Gets Sjögren's Syndrome?

Sjögren's can affect anybody, male or female, young or old, and from any ethnic background. However, if there is such a thing as a "typical" Sjögren's patient, she is probably middle-aged and female. It is common for the disease to develop (or be diagnosed) around the age of forty or over, and it is estimated that only around one in ten patients are male. It is also estimated that around one in every five hundred people has Sjögren's. Nobody is sure why Sjögren's attacks mainly women, but it is possible that female hormones, such as estrogen, are involved in making women more susceptible to the disease.

There is some evidence that a predisposition to Sjögren's may run in families. Other autoimmune diseases—particularly lupus and thyroid problems—are also more common among the relatives of people with Sjögren's.

Scientists are pretty sure that there is a genetic component to Sjögren's syndrome. Genes known as HLA (human leukocyte antigen) genes are involved in controlling the immune response and are inherited, just like the genes for eye color or curly hair. One gene, called HLA-DR3, is frequently found in those of European ancestry who have primary Sjögren's, and different genes are associated with the disorder in other ethnic groups. However, there are likely to be multiple genes involved, and at this stage it is too early to state definitely which particular genes these are.

So, while it may be possible to inherit a genetic predisposition to Sjögren's syndrome, merely having the right combination of genes (and, remember, we don't yet know what they are) does not guarantee you will develop full-blown Sjögren's. Many relatives will test positive for the antibodies present in Sjögren's, but will never develop any of the symptoms.

It is thought that a genetic predisposition alone is not enough to produce the disease, and that there may also have to be a trigger. As yet, scientists are not quite sure what that trigger is, but there is evidence to suggest that—in some cases at least—it may be a viral infection. In my own case, for example, I developed a throat infection shortly before the first symptoms of Sjögren's syndrome manifested themselves. Another sufferer I know developed symptoms after a severe bout of flu. Some researchers have suggested that the Epstein-Barr virus (the cause of glandular fever) may be the culprit, but there is as yet no proof of this. Again, no consistent pattern emerges around the globe. For example, in Japan an illness very similar to Sjögren's is associated with a virus that can cause a rare form of leukemia—the HTLV1 virus—but this association is not found anywhere else. In countries bordering the Mediterranean, a link between the hepatitis C virus and Sjögren's has been observed, but this hasn't been found in other parts of the world.

Preventing Sjögren's

While symptoms are often treatable, there is no way of preventing

Sjögren's syndrome. But early diagnosis and intervention can prevent complications. As already stated in the Introduction, self-help measures can go a long way toward making you more comfortable, while regular medical check-ups can help monitor any changes in symptoms.

Chapter 2

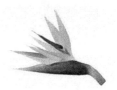

Diagnosing
Sjögren's Syndrome

It can take a long time to get a diagnosis of Sjögren's syndrome, be-cause, as described in the previous chapter, people can display a wide variety of symptoms, which may make it difficult for doctors to arrive at a conclusive diagnosis. One of the great frustrations of Sjögren's is that people look well but feel awful. It is not uncom-mon to take a roundabout route to eventual diagnosis. My own doctor had just prescribed eye-drops for my dry eyes when my den-tist noticed the excessive dryness in my mouth, put two and two together, and sent me off for further tests that eventually resulted in a diagnosis of Sjögren's.

Julia had suffered for several months with various complaints, including aching joints, sore eyes, and sweating attacks. Like many other people, she was referred to the rheumatology department of her local hospital, and she received a subsequent diagnosis of Sjö-gren's only months later.

Another potential complication is that the symptoms that are characteristic of Sjögren's syndrome can also indicate several other illnesses. Even those with Sjögren's may not realize that there is a connection between their gritty eyes and their parched mouths, their itching skin and their joint problems. Some physi-cians may not be very well informed about the condition and may also fail to spot the pattern, instead trying to treat the individual symptoms as separate problems or beginning investigations into other diseases.

A sympathetic doctor may refer a patient to a specialist for one of the problems—perhaps an ophthalmologist for the dry eyes or an ENT consultant for problems with a dry mouth and hoarseness of voice. Or perhaps you yourself may consult your dentist about problems, such as inflamed gums, a dry tongue, or tooth decay.

Your doctor will probably ask you about any other symptoms you may have. An informed doctor may look for other signs of Sjögren's, such as red, itchy eyes; swollen salivary glands; a dry, cracked tongue; and enlarged salivary glands in your neck. You'll also want to discuss what medications you are taking—both prescription and over-the-counter—as many medications can exacerbate oral dryness, notably:

◆ Tricyclic antidepressants

◆ Monoamine oxidase inhibitors

◆ Muscle-relaxing agents

◆ Blood pressure medications

◆ Heart medication

◆ Antiseizure drugs

Once these factors have been eliminated, your doctor may arrange a series of diagnostic tests, including those described below.

The Schirmer I Test

The Schirmer I test is a simple test for dry eyes that indicates whether the lachrymal glands are producing enough tears. A strip of sterile filter paper (a bit like blotting paper) is inserted between the eyeball and the lower eyelid and left there for five minutes. When it is removed, the doctor measures how much of the strip is wet (a normal reading is usually in excess of eight millimeters per five minutes).

Tests Using Dyes

These tests are carried out by eye specialists (ophthalmologists) who use a slit lamp imaging to detect changes. The doctor assesses whether the eye has been damaged by the diminished output of tears by inserting a drop of dye (rose bengal or fluorescein). The dye clings briefly to any dry or damaged areas, making it possible to identify them more easily.

Mouth Examination

The doctor will look into the mouth for signs of dryness and will check to see if any of the main salivary glands (parotid, submandibular, and sublingual) are swollen. Tell-tale signs of dryness include:

- Dry, sticky mouth
- Smooth-looking tongue
- Redness
- Dental decay
- Little, or very thick, saliva
- Dry, cracked lips
- Sores at the corners of the mouth

A simple screening test involves the collection and measurement of the saliva production over a defined period by getting the person to spit all saliva formed into a measuring container. Normally, 1.5 milliliters would be collected in fifteen minutes.

The doctor may also try to stimulate saliva production by massaging the glands or administering a sour substance. Cloudy saliva can indicate the presence of infection.

Saliva manufactured by the parotid glands (the ones that make you look like a hamster when you have mumps) enters the mouth via two tiny openings inside the mouth that are located next to the upper molars on either side. These openings are called

Stenson's ducts. If the doctor wishes to check the flow of saliva, a suction cup can be placed over the opening and the amount of saliva measured.

It is also possible to image the salivary glands using ultrasound, MRI, or radioactive isotopes, but these tests are not commonly used in everyday practice.

Lip Biopsy

To be entirely sure that a patient has Sjögren's syndrome, a lip biopsy may be carried out. Often this procedure is done on an outpatient basis in the oral surgery department of the local hospital. It is a short procedure, during which one of the tiny minor salivary glands is removed from inside the lower lip. It is usually carried out under local anesthetic while the patient sitting up in a dentist's chair.

The gland is then examined in the pathology department, to determine if it is inflamed and whether it has been invaded by lymphocytes (white cells), both indications that Sjögren's syndrome may be present.

Blood Tests

As discussed earlier, blood tests are frequently used to diagnose the condition because Sjögren's patients manufacture specific antibodies in their blood. These tests determine the presence of autoantibodies and immunoglobulins and help doctors to eliminate other possibilities, such as rheumatoid arthritis or lupus.

Autoantibodies

Autoantibodies are antibodies that react to the cells and tissues of the person who produces them.

Antinuclear Antibodies

This family of antibodies is classically found in all patients with lupus but also occur in up to 70 percent of patients with Sjögren's.

Two of the most notable antibodies in this family (as far as Sjögren's patients are concerned)—Ro and La—are particularly important in Sjögren's cases. Other antinuclear antibodies are found in the blood of people with lupus but can also be present in Sjögren's patients—so on their own, their presence does not mean that a patient is suffering from lupus.

Ro and La

Also known as SS-A and SS-B, Ro and La are antinuclear antibodies that are frequently found in the blood of Sjögren's sufferers. Ro antibodies are found in 60–70 percent of patients, while La antibodies are found in around 40 percent, particularly those with primary Sjögren's.

Ro antibodies can also be present in people with other autoimmune disorders, so on their own, they do not necessarily confirm the presence of Sjögren's syndrome. Also, it is possible to have Sjögren's without having these antibodies.

Rheumatoid Factor

This is the name given to a group of antibodies that are found not only in the blood of people with rheumatoid arthritis, but sometimes in people who have other autoimmune diseases, including Sjögren's syndrome. On its own, this factor does not mean that an individual has rheumatoid arthritis. Often it is the finding of both an antinuclear antibody and rheumatoid factor on a screening test that alerts a doctor to the possibility of Sjögren's.

Markers of Inflammation

The most common screening test for Sjögren's measures the erythrocyte sedimentation rate (ESR). The ESR is a nonspecific screening test for various diseases. This one-hour test measures the distance (in millimeters) that red blood cells settle toward the bottom of a specially marked test tube of unclotted blood. A normal result is less than twenty millimeters for women under fifty years old. The sedimentation rate increases if there is inflammation for any reason. If an individual's ESR is high, for example over fifty, it may indicate that that person has Sjögren's syndrome or a connective tissue disease. Interestingly, another frequently measured marker of inflammation, the C reactive protein, is not raised in Sjögren's, so this discrepancy again may suggest Sjögren's.

Immunoglobulins

These are normal antibodies (proteins) that help protect the body from disease. If a person has Sjögren's, her levels are usually high. Levels can vary according to how active a patient's Sjögren's is at any given time, so once you have been diagnosed, your doctor may wish to carry out this test at regular intervals.

Other Tests

In addition to all these blood tests, it is possible that your doctor may wish you to have a chest X ray, because Sjögren's can cause inflammation of the lungs in rare cases. Your doctor may also test your urine to see how well your kidneys are functioning.

Once you are on medication, you will probably have to have regular blood tests to track the progress of your illness and to check that the medicines you are taking are not harming your liver, kidneys, or other organs.

Today, there is a broad international consensus on the diagnosis of Sjögren's syndrome. There is no single diagnostic test and the diagnosis depends upon fulfilling five out of six sets of criteria. Two of these criteria relate to symptoms of dry eyes or mouth, and two more are concerned with evidence of impaired tear or salivary secretion as shown by medical tests, such as the Schirmer I test or tests using dyes. The remaining two are the presence of Ro or La antibodies in the blood and an abnormal lip biopsy.

What Happens Next?

A diagnosis can be reassuring, ending a period of uncertainty and suspense. Now that you have a name to put to your condition, you can start getting to know this illness and the best ways of managing it. This process may be a matter of trial and error, but you can find your way along with advice and help from your doctor. The next chapter looks at some of the treatments available to combat Sjögren's syndrome.

Chapter 3

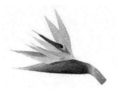

Treating Sjögren's Syndrome — Simple Measures

The simplest treatments are often the most effective, and they are certainly the ones least likely to cause unwanted side effects. It is likely that your doctor or specialist will begin with some of these simple approaches in the hope that the more complex (and potentially more problematic) drug treatments won't become necessary.

Simple Solutions for a Dry Mouth

Xerostomia—the chronic dry mouth characteristic of Sjögren's patients—can be distressing, and in severe cases it can make swallowing unduly difficult. If you choose to use a solution to keep the mouth and throat reasonably moist, make sure its use does not come with harmful side effects, such as dental decay. Sugary sweets and drinks may stimulate the flow of saliva, for instance, but they're hardly a good idea when the downside is rampant cavities and obesity!

Luckily, a variety of sugar-free sweets are now available. Used in moderation, they can be very valuable in stimulating failing saliva glands and increasing production. Sour substances, like lemon and vinegar, also tend to make your mouth water, so it should be no surprise that cider vinegar diluted with water is an old folk remedy for fatigue, arthritis, and every ailment under the sun. Be careful, however, as lemon can cause tooth erosion. Sugarless chewing gum is another good standby and can be chewed throughout the day. And, of course, don't forget plain drinking water, that good, old favorite. If you want to avoid frequent trips to the bathroom, try rinsing your mouth with water, rather than swallowing it.

The standard medical treatment for a dry mouth is artificial saliva, which comes in tubes or spray bottles of either a colorless, slightly sticky gel or as a rather slimy liquid. Some people say that the gel lasts a little longer than the liquid, as it adheres better to the inside of the mouth. Like real saliva, the liquid is liable to be swallowed, but this doesn't really matter, as artificial saliva can be used as many times as needed. Artificial saliva can be prescribed or bought over the counter at your local pharmacy. Products containing fluoride are best.

More Tips for Dry Mouth

- ◆ Avoid eating foods that can dry or irritate your mouth, such as nuts, chocolate, strong cheeses, and shellfish.

- ◆ Soothe dry, cracked lips by using oil- or petroleum-based lip balm or lipstick.

- ◆ Use a mouth rinse, ointment, or gel recommended or provided by your doctor on sore areas to control pain and inflammation.

- ◆ Drink fluids throughout the day and rinse your mouth frequently. Grape juice can be helpful, especially when held in the mouth for a few moments before being swallowed.

- ◆ Suck on ice chips or frozen grapes.

- ◆ Eat a diet rich in raw fruits and vegetables to stimulate the parasympathetic nervous system and reduce acidity in the mouth and stomach. This, in turn, can help stimulate saliva.

♦ Avoid caffeinated teas and coffee, which are diuretic and add to drying. Try weak versions or drink herbal teas instead.

♦ Breathe through the nose, rather than the mouth. A soft cervical collar, used while sleeping, may prevent open-mouth breathing by supporting the jaw.

♦ Sleep in a cool bedroom and avoid air conditioning if possible.

Check Your Mouth

It is a good idea to check your mouth regularly, so that you know what is normal for you and are more likely to notice the development of unusual redness, other coloration, mouth pain, or bleeding. Only a minority of people with a painful or burning mouth will actually develop thrush, a fungal infection characterized by white patches inside the mouth or as red, burning areas in the mouth. However, if you feel you have symptoms of a mouth infection or if your usual symptoms deteriorate and you have a painful mouth and burning tongue, consult your doctor or dentist.

If you develop thrush, you may find that bathing the mouth with live yogurt is soothing. Alternatively, your doctor can prescribe antifungal drugs. These can be taken in tablet form and may take a couple of weeks to work. Various viruses and bacteria can also cause infections, and these can be treated with antiviral or antibiotic medicines.

Oral Hygiene

Julia

I have lost one tooth and am taking great care of the rest! I have gotten to know my dentist and hygienist quite well. They understand my Sjögren's and provide helpful advice on cleaning, check-ups, and so on. So far I've avoided losing any more teeth.

Good oral hygiene is essential for people who have Sjögren's. Saliva contains substances that get rid of the mouth bacteria that cause cavities and infections, so if there is a decrease in saliva levels, problems can develop. Tooth decay is common in Sjögren's, and some people may also suffer mouth infections. Some people find it to be helpful to cultivate a good relationship with their dentist and oral hygienist so they can become more informed about Sjögren's and the effects it can have on the mouth.

- Visit your dentist regularly to have your teeth examined and cleaned. Ask your dentist if you should take fluoride supplements, use a fluoride gel at night, or have a protective varnish put on your teeth to protect the enamel.

- Rinse your mouth with water several times a day. Don't use a mouthwash that contains alcohol, as it causes dryness.

- Brush your teeth immediately before and after eating, as well as before bedtime. Brushing before meals helps to eliminate oral bacteria that might cling to food particles and encourage decay. Electric toothbrushes may be helpful.

- Avoid sticky, sugary foods to reduce the risk of tooth decay. Three teaspoons of sugar eaten once daily is less detrimental to tooth enamel than one teaspoon of sugar eaten at three different times over the course of a day. Every time sugar is eaten, bacteria produce acid for twenty minutes.

- Avoid sugary and acidic foods, including citrus fruits, which can damage tooth enamel. If you do eat or drink them, brush your teeth immediately afterwards.

- Choose sugar-free varieties of soft drinks and use a straw to protect the teeth from acidity.

◆ Prepare a mouthwash solution using a quarter of a teaspoon of baking soda dissolved in a quarter of a cup of warm water to reduce oral acidity and produce a fresh taste in the mouth.

◆ Don't use toothpaste designed for stained teeth because it might be too harsh on your tooth enamel. Use fluoride toothpaste to gently brush your teeth, gums, and tongue.

◆ Floss your teeth every day. Small brushes are also very effective for cleaning between the teeth.

◆ Apply the contents of a vitamin E capsule to your mouth, especially at night.

Simple Solutions for Dry Eyes

Your doctor will probably recommend a simple treatment in the form of artificial tears. Like artificial saliva, this is a product designed to mimic the natural substance as closely as possible; but of course it isn't as effective, because it tends to drain away and then has to be replaced manually. Nevertheless, if you have dry, gritty eyes, artificial tears are an absolute godsend. They can remove the discomfort almost instantly.

Artificial tears can be prescribed or bought over the counter at a pharmacy. They come in two different forms: liquid drops, which come in a squeeze bottle, and gel tears, which come in a small tube. To apply, you simply pull the lower eyelid slightly forward and squeeze a few drops onto the surface of the eye. Blinking will spread the fluid over the eyeball.

The choice of drops or gel is a matter of personal preference, and it may be worth experimenting if one type does not help. I personally like the gel tears, because they last a good, long time. On the down side, they are quite thick and have a tendency to blur the vision for a short while after insertion. Because of this potential for causing blurry vision, they may be more suitable for nighttime use, and using them at this time will lead to less burning, dryness, and itching upon waking in the morning.

Sometimes people become sensitized to the preservative in some artificial tears, which can be a particular problem in people with blocked nasolachrymal ducts. They start to experience stinging in the eyes when the drops are used, and then preservative-free drops are needed.

Other Eye-Protection Tips

♦ Protect your eyes from the wind, hair dryers, air conditioners, heaters, and radiators.

♦ Use goggles when swimming.

♦ Avoid smoky or dusty atmospheres.

♦ Apply mascara only to the tips of your lashes so it doesn't get into your eyes, and put eyeliner or eye shadow only on the skin above your lashes, not on the sensitive skin underneath.

♦ Wear wraparound sunglasses to help protect your eyes from the sun, wind, and dust.

♦ Blink several times a minute while reading or working on the computer.

♦ Avoid rubbing your eyes, however strong the temptation is to do so.

♦ Put a humidifier in the rooms where you spend the most time, including the bedroom, or install a humidifier in your heating and air conditioning unit.

♦ Ask your doctor whether any of your medications contribute to dryness and, if so, how to reduce that effect.

♦ Consider soft contact lenses rather than the traditional hard ones, though many patients with Sjögren's are unable to wear contact lenses at all.

Treating Dry Eye with Petroleum Jelly

The eye's tear film has three layers:

1. A mucin layer next to the eyeball

2. A tear (aqueous) layer on top of the mucin layer

3. A lipid (fatty, oily) layer that prevents the tear layer from evaporating

In Sjögren's syndrome, dry eyes result from problems in both the tear and the lipid layer. Not only do Sjögren's patients produce insufficient tears, their tears also evaporate faster than they should because of an inadequate lipid layer, thereby compounding the problem.

This problem has been tackled in an interesting way with the help of that humble substance, petroleum jelly. According to research by Dr. Donald MacKeen of the Sjögren's Syndrome Foundation, petroleum jelly placed next to the eye helps reduce dryness and the blink rates of patients. This so-called *supracutaneous* effect is due to the fact that the jelly gradually spreads, or migrates, into the surrounding eyeskin, supposedly reducing soreness and dryness.

A controlled study reported in the *British Journal of Ophthalmology* tested this theory. Researchers Dr. Kazuo Tsubota and colleagues of the Tokyo Dental College found that participants reported significant improvement in dry eye symptoms when calcium carbonate in a petroleum ointment was applied to the lower eyelids.

From anecdotal reports, it also appears that petroleum jelly causes less burning and less tearing of the skin around the eye and lessens the need for artificial tears, goggles, or protective glasses—though you may look a little shiny around the eye! For best results, use 100-percent pure petroleum.

If you try this treatment, here are some tips:

◆ Start off with a small blob of jelly and don't apply too near the eye—a little outside the lashline is as close as you should get.

◆ Use a cotton swab or clean finger to apply.

◆ Treat both upper and lower lids, applying an extra amount at bedtime and during the night.

◆ Expect some blurring. It may be best to experiment with this at bedtime.

Simple Solutions for Aches and Pains

Joint pain can be a fact of life for people with Sjögren's. The good news is that over-the-counter painkillers can be used to very good effect in many cases. The main nonprescription analgesics are acetaminophen, combinations of acetaminophen and codeine, and ibuprofen.

Ibuprofen is an anti-inflammatory drug that is particularly good for arthritic-type pain, although acetaminophen is generally kinder on the stomach. If you suffer from stomach trouble (ulcers, gastritis, bleeding), check with your doctor to make sure that it is all right for you to take these types of drugs.

You can also buy pain-relieving creams and gels based on ibuprofen and other anti-inflammatory drugs, such as ibuprofen gel, ibuprofen and codeine gel, and diclofenac sodium (Voltaren) emulgel. These gels are effective for treating localized pain, such as a sore shoulder or knee. The concentration of the drug that reaches the individual trouble spot is much greater if gel is rubbed on the skin than if a painkiller is taken orally.

Again, these products are available without a prescription, but your doctor may also prescribe them for you. It is worth establishing whether the cost of the prescription would be higher than the cost of buying the drug over the counter.

Simple Solutions for Skin Problems

To treat dry skin, apply heavy moisturizing creams and ointments three or four times a day to trap moisture in the skin. Lotions, which are lighter than creams and ointments, aren't recommended because they evaporate quickly and can actually contribute to dry skin.

Take quick showers (less than five minutes), use a moisturizing soap, pat your skin almost dry, and then cover it with a cream or ointment at once. If you prefer a bath, add some emollient oil and then soak yourself in it for a few minutes to give your skin time to absorb moisture. Avoid prolonged hot showers or baths.

Other Tips for Skin Problems

◆ Talk to your health-care professional about using emollients containing salicylic acid, lactate, or urea for particularly dry patches of skin. For itching, your doctor might recommend that you use a skin cream or ointment containing steroids.

◆ Place a humidifier (and an air purifier, if you feel it helps) in your home and at work to increase your comfort by keeping the humidity in your surroundings between 30 and 50 percent. You may want to use a humidifier year-round. Some experts advise using a cool-mist, ultrasonic humidifier; be sure to clean it daily.

◆ Use a nasal rinse or spray made of water and salt to alleviate a dry nose and nasal congestion.

◆ Consider using a soft cervical collar while you sleep to discourage your mouth from opening, since an open mouth can contribute to nasal and airway dryness.

◆ Use moisturizing skin creams or ointments throughout the day.

- Use only moisturizing soaps while bathing and avoid antibacterial soaps or abrasive cleansers.

- Don't dry your skin completely after bathing. Leave a film of moisture and then moisturize with a cream or ointment. Emollients with urea, lactate, or salicylic acid help in sloughing off dead skin and allowing a healthier, softer skin to emerge.

- Cover your skin and head when outside, use a sunscreen with a sun protection factor (SPF) of 15 or higher, and try to avoid being in the sun for long periods of time.

- Coat your lips with petroleum-based lubricants or certain lipsticks to prevent drying.

- Consider installing a water conditioner if you live in a hard-water area.

- Talk to your health-care professional about discontinuing your use of decongestants and antihistamines because they dry your mouth and nasal areas.

- If you suffer from nosebleeds or sinus problems, try using a saline nasal wash (a mixture of water and salt that you can prepare at home).

Simple Solutions for Other Problem Areas

Vaginal Dryness

Vaginal dryness may be one of the more embarrassing effects of Sjögren's syndrome. Indeed, some women may fail to be diagnosed because they assume it is a symptom of menopause that they have to put up with. A vaginal moisturizing product or lubricant may help relieve discomfort. Sustained use of lubricants can, however, disrupt the normal mucosa of the vagina, making lubricants inappropriate for long-term application. Instead, vitamin E suppositories may be helpful. During the first month of use, insert the suppository into the vagina once a day; after several months, one suppository one to three times a week may be enough.

Swollen Glands

A swollen face and jaw, and sometimes toothache and headache, are common symptoms of an inflamed gland. If you suffer from these, try massaging the swollen gland and applying heat. Sucking on hard sugarless sweets may also help.

Cold Extremities

Some people with Sjögren's suffer cold hands and feet due to impaired circulation. In particular, some may suffer from Raynaud's syndrome, a spasm of the arteries that causes the fingers and toes to go numb and turn white. This reaction often takes place in cold-weather conditions. Keep gloves handy for cold jobs like removing items from the fridge and freezer or going outside into the garden. Thermal mitts and socks may help. A warm hat is also helpful to help retain heat in the body.

Inflamed Vocal Cords

People with Sjögren's can develop hoarseness if their vocal cords become inflamed or irritated from throat dryness or coughing. To prevent further strain on your vocal cords, try not to clear your throat before speaking. Instead, take a sip of water, chew gum, or suck on candy. To help get sound out, make an 'h' sound, hum, or laugh to gently bring the vocal cords together. Clearing your throat does the same thing, but since it's hard on the vocal cords and causes further irritation, you should avoid this practice.

Chapter 4

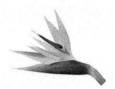

Treatments for Sjögren's

Unfortunately, there isn't as yet any cure for Sjögren's. The objective of conventional treatment is to control symptoms, individually or collectively. The good news is that for most patients—particularly those with primary Sjögren's—treatment works well and doesn't cause too many side effects.

Although most Sjögren's patients are looked after by a rheumatologist, all kinds of practitioners from different specialties may be involved in your treatment, including:

- A dentist
- An oral surgeon
- An ear, nose, and throat (ENT) specialist
- An ophthalmologist (eye specialist)
- An orthoptist (professional who deals with abnormal eye movements)
- A pain relief specialist

Although it can be beneficial to draw on the skills and perspectives of different practitioners, I sometimes think that, with so many different specialists involved, things can get unnecessarily complicated and wires can become crossed. In my own case, for example, I have seen all of the above at one time or another; but when I have suddenly become acutely ill, nobody has been quite sure which department I come under or who ought to decide whether I should be admitted to the hospital—and if so, to which ward!

It would be ideal if all the medical professionals involved in your care could meet and discuss the different symptoms and problems together. Or, even better, if there could be dedicated Sjögren's clinics all over the country, where professionals from different disciplines could work together closely and exchange information on patients. Until that day, the best you can do is to inform yourself about your condition so that you can approach the right professional, for the right treatment, at the right time.

More Complex Medication

Over-the-counter products are all an important part of the anti-Sjögren's medicine cabinet, and most patients use at least some of them on a regular basis. But when symptoms are worse than the odd bit of grittiness in the eye, the slightly dry mouth, or the occasional twinge in a joint, doctors have access to much more powerful forms of treatment. The negative side of these drugs is that they are liable to produce more undesirable side effects than simpler, nonprescription remedies.

Dry Mouth

Some prescription drugs, like pilocarpine, stimulate increased salivary flow. Pilocarpine has been shown to be effective in clinical trials with patients who still have some function in their salivary glands. It doesn't suit everybody, however, because some people develop side effects, such as sweating, urinary frequency, dizziness, and flushing. These effects can often be overcome by starting on a small dose, increasing the dose gently over a period of weeks, and stopping on a less than maximal dose if necessary. How useful it is on an individual basis is best determined by trying it and seeing whether or not it works.

It is worth mentioning again that there are some drugs that can make a dry mouth worse. Your doctor should research everything you are taking to ensure that you are not contributing to your own condition. Examples of drugs that may make oral dryness worse are antidepressants, tricyclic analgesics (such as amitryptiline), antihistamines, and beta blockers.

Other Oral Problems

As we've seen, fungal infections and dental cavities are common problems when the mouth is dry. Another hazard for those with Sjögren's is the possibility of infections or blockages in the major saliva glands.

I once developed a very strange bulge under my tongue. When I lifted my tongue, it looked as if I had a pink glassy bauble on the floor of my mouth. It turned out that this bulge was the result of a blocked sublingual gland that had to be surgically removed. It is a good idea to remove a blocked gland of this type because there is always a slight chance of malignancy, but in most cases—like mine—it is a simple calcium deposit, caused by a thickening of the saliva.

When the saliva glands become infected—particularly the parotid glands at the sides of the face and neck—they tend to become sore and swell up, causing a person to look as if she has the mumps. The saliva may also become thick and infected. If this happens, a course of antibiotics will probably put things in order quite quickly. Only in rare cases do glands have to be removed.

Inflammation

Inflammation in the body increases when Sjögren's becomes more active, and nonsteroidal anti-inflammatory drugs (NSAIDs) are among the most commonly used drugs to combat this inflammation. NSAIDs don't just reduce inflammation (as in arthritis); they also reduce pain. In many ways they are similar to aspirin and ibuprofen, and so their side effects are also similar. In particular, there is a risk of stomach irritation and/or bleeding. In severe cases, sensitive patients could even develop a peptic ulcer. Some people cannot tolerate NSAIDs, but most can, especially with careful use and the help of drugs like lansoprazole (Prevacid) and celecoxib (Celebrex) that protect the stomach. Over-the-counter remedies, such as Gaviscon, can also help.

Suppositories reduce the chance of stomach problems as well. I know many people turn green at the very thought of a suppository, but I use diclofenac (Voltaren) suppositories, and, believe me, they're a godsend. They get the drug into the bloodstream more quickly than tablets and do not have such an irritating effect on the stomach.

Overactive Immune System

Sjögren's is very much a disorder of the immune system—an overactive immune system, in fact. One of the ways doctors treat it, then, is to try to suppress that overactivity.

The first line of immunosuppressant medication is steroids. The most commonly prescribed steroid is prednisolone, which is generally given in tablet form but can be administered by drip if you are in a hospital and the dose is a large one. Like NSAIDs, steroids can have an irritating effect on the stomach, so they are often prescribed in the form of enteric-coated tablets. This coating does not dissolve until the tablet is safely out of the stomach and into the intestine.

Steroids are of help to some, but they are strong drugs that have undesirable side effects. If possible, it is better to use them just for flare-ups, rather than continuously. Long-term use can lead to such diverse problems as osteoporosis, peptic ulcer, diabetes, fragile skin, poor wound healing, and eye troubles.

There is also the problem that everyone immediately thinks of when steroids are mentioned: weight gain. Putting on huge amounts of weight isn't inevitable, but the fact that steroids increase the appetite doesn't exactly help! They also promote water retention and tend to produce a plump, round-faced appearance that can be embarrassing. I know I've struggled with my weight since I started on steroids and would dearly love not to have to take them. But unfortunately, every time the dose is reduced I have another flare-up. So for the time being at least I'm just grateful that there's something I can take to ease the pain.

Eating sensibly is very important—not just because of the risk of weight gain, but also to guard against bone problems. Your doctor can advise you on a good, bone-strengthening diet with lots of calcium and green vegetables, but you may also wish to take a mineral supplement specifically designed to promote bone health. Today, most doctors will also prescribe some form of therapy to help you avoid osteoporosis if you are likely to be taking steroids for more than a few weeks. The commonly used agents are bisphosphonate drugs or calcium and vitamin D compounds. Women who are past menopause or who—like me—have had their ovaries removed may be wise to take some form of treatment to protect their bones. Your doctor will help you determine what is the right course of action for you.

The more powerful immunosuppressant drugs, such as azathioprine, cyclosporin, and methotrexate, do not help Sjögren's. Antirheumatic medication generally does not help either, with the exception of hydroxychloroquine, which provides some modest benefit in improving fatigue and joint pain, according to laboratory tests. It is very slow acting, and people may need to take it for six months before seeing any benefit.

Chronic Pain

Of course, specific anti-inflammatory or immunosuppressant medication cannot always solve the problem, and some people will be left with some degree of chronic pain. Others may have periodic flare-ups when things seem to get out of control and the pain starts taking over. When this happens, your local pain clinic and pain specialists can help.

Unlike acute pain, chronic (long-lasting) pain can't easily be wiped out with a couple of painkillers. The messages between the brain and the nerves can become garbled, and other medication may work more efficiently in sorting this out. Some of the drugs commonly used in pain clinics are the following:

- Gabapentin (Neurontin), originally an antiepilepsy drug, but found to be an effective pain suppressant

- Carbamazepine (Tegretol)

- Amitriptyline (Elavil), an old-style tricyclic antidepressant that is effective for pain but that worsens dryness of the eyes and mouth

Your pain specialist may also use a range of other techniques and treatments. We'll look at these in Chapter 6.

Medications to Avoid If Possible

Several types of medication can cause dryness or allergic reactions and can make your symptoms worse. Talk to your health professional if you are taking any of the following medications:

- Some blood pressure medications

- Antidepressants

- Antihistamines

- Decongestants

- Diuretics

- Muscle spasm medications

- Bladder medications

- Some heart medicines

- Parkinson's disease medications

It is important, however, to not abruptly halt any course of treatment and to continue taking any of these medications until you are advised to stop by your health-care professional.

Surgery

One way to relieve dry eyes is to undergo a minor surgical procedure to seal the tear ducts that drain tears from your eyes (punctal occlusion). Collagen or silicone plugs are inserted into the ducts for a temporary closure. Collagen plugs eventually dissolve, but silicone plugs will keep the ducts sealed until they fall out or are removed. Your doctor may use a laser to permanently seal your ducts.

Acupuncture

According to traditional Chinese medicine, disease is the result of stagnant *qi* (pronounced "chee"), the vital energy of the body, which in turn affects organ function. Acupuncturists stimulate and balance the flow of qi by inserting hair-thin needles into specific points in the body along energy pathways called meridians. Unlike many conventional medications, acupuncture has no known side effects. In fact, treatments release pain-fighting endorphins.

Studies on the efficacy of acupuncture are few and far between, especially with regard to Sjögren's. Nevertheless, some studies suggest that acupuncture may offer some improvement for the symptoms of dry eyes and dry mouth. One study of people with dry mouth, for example, found that the salivary flow rate improved significantly after six months of acupuncture treatment. The study recommended that, like other forms of alternative medicine, acupuncture is best used as a complement to conventional treatment.

Chapter 5

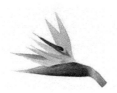

Supplements

Even though there is no cure for Sjögren's at the moment, conventional medicine is a very important means for controlling the disorder and making you more comfortable. Supplements, such as specific vitamins or herbs, can also be helpful for some symptoms.

Vitamins and Minerals

You may be tempted to try treating your Sjögren's with supplements, though this is still something of a lottery. Because research on the benefits of supplements is still limited, individual trial and error—with the approval of your doctor—may be necessary before you find a supplement that meets your needs.

A study of people with Sjögren's by Dr. Gloria Gilbère of the Naturopathic Health and Research Center in Idaho found that many of them were deficient in zinc, as well as vitamin A, vitamin B-6, potassium, and calcium. Generally, however, not much information is available on how specific vitamin or mineral supplements may help in Sjögren's syndrome. Whole foods are always the best sources for vitamins and minerals, but a daily multivitamin may be worthwhile, especially if you tend to limit your diet due to mouth discomfort.

The following vitamins and minerals may help address some of Sjögren's most common symptoms:

- *Vitamin* C protects against inflammation and infection, and it may help protect against dental cavities. Chewable vitamin C, however, is best avoided because it is highly acidic and may damage tooth enamel. Good sources are citrus fruits, berries, tomatoes, cauliflower, potatoes, green leafy vegetables, and peppers.

- *Vitamin* B-6 helps with the functioning of the central nervous system and promotes good skin condition. It's probably best taken as part of a vitamin B compound to avoid creating imbalances with the other B vitamins. Good food sources are fish, bananas, chicken, pork, whole grains, and dried beans.

- *Riboflavin* (vitamin B-2) may offer relief to people who feel as if grit or sand is irritating the inside of the eyelid. B-2 helps with cell growth and respiration; is beneficial to the skin, nails, hair, connective tissues, and sensitive lips and tongues; and is essential for eye health. Lack of it causes itching and irritation of the eyes, lips, and skin. Good sources include milk, liver, yeast, cheese, green leafy vegetables, and fish.

- *Vitamin* E is a good lubricant and, in oil form (some capsules contain oil), can be used around the nose, inside the nose, and inside the mouth. It's found in wheatgerm, soy beans, vegetable oils, broccoli, leafy green vegetables, wholegrains, peanuts, and eggs.

- *Zinc* may help alleviate the decreased taste and smell suffered by some people with Sjögren's. Good sources include oysters, offal, meat, mushrooms, eggs, whole-grain products (including cereals such as oatmeal), and brewer's yeast.

- *Vitamin* A may be useful for dry eyes. A severe vitamin A deficiency can cause dry eyes, and some people with Sjögren's have tried beta-carotene and vitamin-A eye drops.

However, medical authorities caution that the dryness caused by vitamin A deficiency is different from the dry eyes of Sjögren's syndrome, so this sort of supplementation may not be beneficial. As too much vitamin A can cause liver damage, it may be best to eat foods rich in vitamin A instead, such as fish-liver oil, butter, carrots, green leafy vegetables, egg yolks, milk products, and yellow fruits.

◆ *Potassium* is important for healthy cell function, and good sources include fresh fruit and vegetables, especially bananas, dried apricots, pulses (e.g., lentils, peas, beans), mushrooms, potatoes, and spinach.

◆ *Calcium* is critical to healthy bones and teeth, as well as the heart, nervous system, and muscle growth and contraction. It is found in milk and other dairy products, dark green leafy vegetables, canned fish such as salmon and sardines (if you eat the bones), nuts and seeds (almond, brazil, sesame seed), tofu, dried fruit, hard water, flour, and bread (most of which is fortified with calcium).

Other Supplements

Other supplements—from herbs to homeopathic remedies—have been used to relieve symptoms like dry mouth and fatigue. Experiment with the following:

◆ Coenzyme Q10 and L-carnitine green barley are recommended for fatigue.

◆ The herb goldenseal (*Hydrastis canadensis*) can be used as an antibacterial mouthwash. Dissolve thirty drops of goldenseal in two fluid ounces of warm water and swish it around in the mouth to help get rid of bacteria.

◆ Multiflora rose (*Rosa multiflora*) is used in China to moisten a dry mouth. A tea may be made by adding two to four teaspoons of multiflora rose to a cup of boiling water.

- LongoVital is an herbal supplement enriched with the recommended daily doses of vitamins that may have a beneficial and prolonged effect on saliva flow.

- Evening primrose oil is a good source of omega-3 fatty acids that may help relieve both inflammation and dry eyes after several months of use. It acts by correcting imbalances in the immune system, boosting activity in the saliva and tear glands, and increasing PGE1, a beneficial prostaglandin.

- Homeopathic remedies, such as nutmeg (*Nux moschata*), barberry (*Berberis vulgaris*), and hops (*Bryonia*), have been recommended for individuals with dry mouth. Consult a homeopathic physician regarding dosage and regimen.

- Red pepper (capsicum) stimulates salivation and tears. Use it with discretion in cooking, not raw and by itself!

Glucosamine and Chondroitin Sulfate

These supplements are frequently taken to relieve the symptoms of arthritis and are regarded by many as "natural" because they occur naturally in the human body. The pain relief from these supplements is said to be similar to that obtained by taking the milder NSAIDs, such as ibuprofen and aspirin.

Glucosamine is believed to help with the repair of cartilage, while chondroitin sulfate helps to increase its elasticity. Most users find that they experience full benefits within a few months. If a supplement hasn't helped you by then, it probably won't.

Possible Problems with Taking Glucosamine and Chondroitin Sulfate

- Those with shellfish allergies should beware of glucosamine, because it is extracted from crab, shrimp, and lobster shells.

- Side effects may include loose stools and flatulence.

- Pregnant women and those intending to become pregnant shouldn't use these supplements.

- Diabetics who are taking glucosamine need to check their blood sugar more frequently.

- Chondroitin sulfate may thin the blood—an important consideration for anyone using a blood-thinning drug like heparin, warfarin, or daily aspirin.

What to Consider when Choosing a Supplement

- How long will you have to take it before you can expect to experience some benefit?

- Is it likely to interact adversely with your prescribed medication? If so, please do not try it without first consulting your doctor, and don't come off your usual medication without your doctor's agreement.

- Are there any known side effects or dangers?

- Do you know any other people with Sjögren's who have tried it, and did it do them any good?

- Is it manufactured by a reputable company? Buying supplements on the Internet, for example, is a risky business. It might not be the real thing, it might be adulterated, and at best it may be a different strength from that stated on the bottle.

- Are you already taking a supplement? It is best not to take more than one supplement at a time. If you do, check with your doctor to make sure the combination is safe. Just because something is advertised as "natural" does not mean it cannot also be potent and dangerous!

- Are you sure it's safe? Don't take anything unless you're satisfied that it's safe—particularly if you have some other

medical condition (e.g., diabetes, heart problems) that
might complicate matters or if you are pregnant (or intend
to be).

Possible Drug Interactions of Common Supplements

Bromelain	May increase effects of blood-thinning drugs and tetracycline antibiotics.
Echinacea	May counteract immunosuppressant drugs such as glucocorticoids taken for lupus and rheumatoid arthritis. May increase side effects of methotrexate.
Evening primrose oil	Can counteract the effects of anticonvulsant drugs.
Fish oil	May increase effects of blood-thinning drugs and herbs.
Folic acid	Interferes with methotrexate; ask your doctor how to take it.
Gamma-linolenic acid (GLA)	May increase effects of blood-thinning drugs and herbs.
Garlic	Can increase effects of blood-thinning drugs and herbs.
Ginger	Can increase NSAID side effects and effects of blood-thinning drugs and herbs.
Ginkgo	May increase effects of blood-thinning drugs and herbs.
Ginseng	May increase effects of blood-thinning drugs, estrogens, and glucocorticoids; shouldn't be used by those with diabetes; may interact with MAO inhibitors (used in certain antidepressants).
Kava kava	Can increase effects of alcohol, sedatives, and tranquilizers.
Magnesium	May interact with blood-pressure medications.
St John's wort	May enhance effects of narcotics, alcohol, and antidepressants; may increase risk of sunburn; may interfere with iron absorption.
Valerian	Can increase the effects of sedatives and tranquilizers.
Zinc	Can interfere with glucocorticoids and other immunosuppressant drugs.

Chapter 6

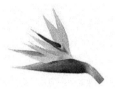

Managing Flare-Ups and Pain

Everybody with Sjögren's has flare-ups, and some also experience pain, especially in the joints. This chapter offers ideas on how to manage these two problems.

Managing Flare-Ups

Even if you function well most of the time or if medication usually controls your illness, you are likely to experience flare-ups. They don't mean you're a failure! In fact, flare-ups can serve a purpose—however unwelcome—in signalling that your body has had enough for the moment and needs some time off. The trick is to try and catch yourself before you reach the "flare" point. Try to get to know your own warning signs—perhaps sudden increased fatigue, achiness, depression, irritability, or just a feeling of being under the weather. Try to get extra rest before you develop a problem.

Taking care of yourself and pacing yourself will help you cut down on the number of flare-ups you have. The causes of your flare-ups may vary, but common ones include the following:

◆ Stress

◆ Fatigue

- Overwork

- Changes in routine

- Certain foods

It may help to keep a diary for a while so that you can spot the triggers and identify the warning signs that may precede a flare-up.

Kimberley found that, with care, she could lead a normal, if sedate, life. However, she had a tendency to speed up and take on too much when she felt well. She would pay heavily for this at times, becoming immobilized with fatigue and joint pain for two or three days, especially in her elbows, feet, knees, and neck. Her warning sign was irritation with her children and with shop assistants! She gradually learned to pay attention to her body's messages before reaching this point and to take more rest along the way.

Laura would have regular flare-ups once a month that were associated with premenstrual syndrome. She experienced dry eyes, shivers, and flu-like symptoms, and she generally felt miserable, wanting only to huddle up in bed with a hot-water bottle. She was extremely thirsty, so she drank—and retained—a great deal of fluid, making her gain several pounds that she lost once her period began. Her other symptoms also eased off during the first two days of her period.

Julia worked from home and so could control her routine to a large extent. She swam three times a week—gently—and generally had a good balance of work and rest. However, she found that eating too much wheat (she loved pasta and French bread) and dairy products and not enough fresh produce, combined with stress, would result in her becoming exhausted and cause a return of symptoms, such as a sore mouth and eyes. Constipation was another warning sign, due to too much refined flour and not enough liquids or high-fiber foods. In the aftermath of a flare-up, she would take a complete break and restock the cupboard and fridge with fruit, vegetables, and whole grains.

What to Do if You Have a Flare-Up: An Action Plan

Drawing up an action plan can help minimize the distress of a flare-up even if you can't totally prevent it. You may find it helpful to stock up with what you need to help deal with flare-ups, such as medication, hot and cold packs, pillows, artificial tears and saliva, and pain-relieving gel (if you find it useful).

If a Flare-Up Strikes

- *Deal with the pain.* Draw on some tried-and-true remedies for alleviating pain, such as medication, a hot-water bottle, a warm bath or shower, or simply lying in bed. Warm compresses or heating pads can help ease joint or gland pain. Be careful not to use pain-relieving gel while taking NSAIDs by mouth, or you may accidentally overdose.

- *Get comfortable.* Call a halt to all activity as much as possible and just rest. Use whatever simple comfort remedies suit you best, such as sucking ice cubes or frozen grapes to help reduce the pain of a dry, cracked mouth (see Chapter 3).

- *Minimize stress.* Now is not the time to engage in a tussle with the bank, to go on a big shopping trip, or to invite your in-laws over. Be kind to yourself and quietly avoid as many sources of stress as possible.

- *Inform your employer.* Employers vary in how understanding they are towards a person with chronic sickness, but try to keep your employer as well informed as possible about your condition.

- *Enlist the help of your family.* Without making a huge fuss, many Sjögren's people appreciate it if the family can take over when a flare-up strikes, giving help with everyday tasks, such as cleaning, laundry, shopping, and so on.

◆ *Look at your balance of exercise and rest.* Maintain your fitness *and* recharge your batteries. If flare-ups are frequent, are you doing too much? Gentle exercise, several times a day, is far better for you than infrequent bursts of over-activity, which are more likely to prompt another flare-up.

◆ *Look at your balance of work and leisure.* If you are having frequent flare-ups, could a change of hours or even of jobs help? Easier said than done, I know, but worthy of consideration if you are having more than your fair share of flare-ups!

Managing Pain

Joint pain is a recognized symptom of Sjögren's, while a few unlucky sufferers sometimes feel aches and pains throughout their entire bodies. Other people's experience may be more idiosyncratic—one Finnish study looked at foot pain as a symptom of Sjögren's!

However, many people with full-blown Sjögren's are also holding down demanding jobs and living a full life on top of that, with pain—if any—limited to the mild discomfort of slightly dry eyes or a shortage of saliva. A study from the National Institutes of Health found that only a minority of people (7 percent) suffered widespread pain due to Sjögren's. Other people may lead a full life most of the time but be swamped by profound fatigue and/or aches and pains if they overreach their personal limits and try to do too much. Still others may experience pain, which may be mild and short-term or more severe and more persistent. So, because each person will have an individual experience of his or her disease, any therapies will need to be tailored to particular problems.

From a physical perspective, having pain in a certain part of the body often makes people reluctant to use that particular joint or group of muscles. As a result, they suffer from muscle weakness and bad posture—which, of course, cause further discomfort. A loss of muscle tone and an overall lack of fitness is a major factor in chronic pain, so improving your general physical condition can make a big difference in the way you feel. Exercise is also well known to boost production of endorphins, the body's natural pain-relieving hormones. (See Chapter 8 for more on exercise.)

The Pain Mechanism

Pain is the body's response to an unpleasant stimulus. When you bang your head or burn your finger, specialized nerve endings detect what is happening and relay pain messages to the peripheral nervous system. This in turn sends messages along the nerve pathways to the central nervous system (the spinal cord and brain).

Scientific research suggests that these pain signals have to reach a threshold before they are relayed. This is known as the "pain gate" theory, as if a certain level of signal opens a gate and lets the pain through. Only when the gate is open do we feel pain. Modern pain clinics can teach patients ways of closing the gate and reducing the pain they experience.

After the unpleasant stimulus has gone, a part of the brain called the thalamus should send out a signal telling the pain to stop. Most of the time this happens, but sometimes the system goes wrong and the pain persists as chronic pain.

Within the brain and nervous system, certain chemicals called neurotransmitters are produced. Some kinds of neurotransmitters—for example serotonin and norepinephrine—seem to be able to decrease pain signals by making the pain sensors release endorphins, the body's natural painkillers.

Although we tend to think of pain as a purely physical thing, in reality it is closely bound up with our psychological well being. If you are depressed, for instance, you are likely to feel greater pain than if you are optimistic and happy. People who have been brought up to ignore pain as much as possible generally feel it less intensely than those who associate pain with great distress and suffering.

So if we want to reduce the amount of pain we feel we need to

- get the body to produce more endorphins
- think positively

Different Types of Pain

There is more than one kind of pain. In fact, there are three main types:

1. Acute This kind of pain is temporary and lessens as an injury heals or a condition abates. It is generally directly related to tissue damage.

2. Chronic Malignant People suffering from various forms of cancer experience this type of pain.

3. Chronic Nonmalignant This pain persists, even after a flare-up has died down, and it is common among sufferers from Sjögren's and FM (fibromyalgia). Somehow, the nervous system stops acting normally and starts generating nothing but pain, even though no further damage is being done to the body. It has been described as a sort of memory of pain. It has no purpose, as it is not protecting the body.

Some chronic pain results from damage to nerve fibers—for example after an attack of shingles—and is called neuropathic pain. Again, these damaged nerves persist in sending out pain messages even though there is no continuing tissue damage.

Chronic pain can range from mild to agonizing and very disabling. Even if it is not severe, the fact that it is there all the time can wreak havoc with sufferers' lives, leading to a feeling of loss of control. This in turn leads to depression, which leads to more pain. It is important to treat acute pain quickly and effectively, because it may develop into chronic pain.

Help from Your Doctor

If you suffer chronic or long-term pain, you may need professional help. The first thing to establish is *why* the pain is present. The approach for eye discomfort due to lack of tears is very different from the widespread muscle pains experienced by those who have a combination of Sjögren's and FM.

See your doctor if you are experiencing pain that you cannot control by your own efforts. Doctors are better than ever before at controlling pain and helping people regain control of their lives, and this may be particularly important if you also suffer from another or associated condition, such as arthritis or FM. For many patients with Sjögren's syndrome, fatigue is the major problem; for others, pain may be the dominant problem, particularly if features of FM are also present. This combination is notoriously difficult to treat, and specialist pain clinics may help.

Pain Clinics and Pain Management Programs

Depending on which facilities are available locally, your family doctor may be able to refer you to someone who specializes in pain management if your case is severe. Some areas may have access to a specialist pain clinic with a multidisciplinary approach to treating pain or a local physician with a special interest in pain relief. Many pain consultants are anesthesiologists, who have a comprehensive knowledge of all methods of pain control, from medication to physiotherapy, nerve blocks to acupuncture. Other professionals may also be involved from a range of disciplines, such as physiotherapy, occupational therapy, clinical psychology, counseling, relaxation therapy, specialist nursing, and acupuncture. Clinical psychologists are often included because the perception of pain is strongly influenced by your state of mind.

Pain management programs can help with chronic pain, and the aim of such programs is usually to break the cycle of pain, loss of fitness, and depression. You can be referred to a pain management program either by your doctor or by a pain clinic. As with a pain clinic, sessions may be taught by a multidisciplinary team made up of doctors, nurses, physiotherapists, occupational therapists, clinical psychologists, and pain specialists. Programs may cover a wide range of topics, many of which can be practiced at home, including:

◆ *Relaxation techniques.* It is surprisingly easy to learn how to relax. Relaxation reduces muscle tension, lessens anxiety, and eases pain (see Chapter 7 for more on relaxation).

◆ *Occupational therapy.* This therapy helps you to find practical ways of doing daily tasks that may be difficult or impossible (e.g., household activities, such as ironing, mowing the lawn, or vacuuming). This therapy helps you to gradually get back into life and work, while increasing morale and reducing pain. Occupational therapists also emphasize the importance of pacing yourself. If you do too much one day, you will pay for it with pain the next. It is far better to ration the amount you do per day, because you will probably get more done in the long run.

◆ *Physiotherapy and exercise.* Even though you may feel incapable of staggering down the road to the post office, the benefits of stretching, strengthening, and aerobic exercise are undeniable. And you will soon realize that—with care and determination—anyone can exercise. If I can do it, you certainly can! Slow stretches relax muscles and ease tension, and low-impact exercise like walking, swimming, and cycling is ideal for building up strength, general fitness, and flexibility (see Chapter 8 for more on exercise). Don't forget that exercise helps to release those pain-relieving endorphins too! The golden rule is: Don't do too much too quickly. Ease into any activity gradually or you may do more harm than good.

◆ *Counseling/family therapy.* Counseling helps to relieve pain because it can improve your outlook and thought patterns. Some courses include a session for partners and other family members to help increase their understanding and ease relationship problems. When the course finishes, you can continue the benefits by having follow-up meetings, joining a support group, or becoming involved in on-line discussion forums (see Resources).

Pain Medication

Medication, while important, is not always the be-all-and-end-all of pain control, and stronger medication may not control your pain more effectively than one that is less strong.

Timing is important, and most drugs need to be taken at set intervals for maximum effectiveness. It may be that regular, moderate doses of a medium-strength analgesic are more useful in controlling your pain than less well-timed doses of stronger medication.

Pain clinics use a wide variety of pills and potions. Not all of them were designed originally as pain-relieving drugs.

Types of Common Pain Medications for Sjögren's	
NSAIDs	Nonsteroidal anti-inflammatory drugs. Over-the-counter varieties include ibuprofen and aspirin.
Acetaminophen	Good at controlling pain and fever, but less effective at combating inflammation.
Narcotics	Generally the last resort in terms of analgesia. Although recent research suggests that drugs like morphine are not necessarily addictive when used to combat pain, doctors are still reluctant to prescribe them except in cases of terminal illness.
Antidepressants	Older types of antidepressants, such as amitriptyline (Elavil), can be useful in treating chronic pain. They are nonaddictive but can have side effects.
Anticonvulsants	Some drugs originally designed for the treatment of epilepsy, like gabapentin (Neurontin) and carbamazepine (Tegretol), are effective in treating chronic nerve pain.
Corticosteroids	Drugs like prednisolone are very good at reducing inflammation and swelling, but they do have potentially serious side effects.

Types of Common Pain Medications for Sjögren's (cont'd.)

Tramadol	A synthetic analgesic used mainly for chronic pain, but also sometimes to treat acute pain.
Capsaicin	A topical cream derived from chili peppers. When it is applied to the skin, there is an initial burning sensation. It is believed to work by interrupting pain signals.

Chapter 7

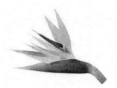

How to Help Yourself — Lifestyle Issues

Being involved in your own care is really important in Sjögren's syndrome. Experts believe taking some amount of control can have a beneficial effect on your overall well-being and quality of life. Besides, with a condition like Sjögren's that has such a variety of symptoms, being involved yourself is often the most effective way of dealing with those symptoms. This chapter looks at lifestyle issues that can help, such as getting plenty of rest, eating well, and doing mild exercise daily.

Fatigue

Tiredness is probably the leading complaint in people with Sjögren's syndrome. It may take different forms and can have more than one cause depending on whether or not you have another condition as well as Sjögren's.

Some experts describe two sorts of fatigue in Sjögren's syndrome:

1. *Late morning or early afternoon fatigue.* You get up full of energy but tend to run out of steam later in the day. This is sometimes called *inflammatory fatigue.* People suffering from this type tend to report flu-like symptoms.

2. *Morning fatigue.* You get up feeling you have not had a proper night's rest because your sleep has been disrupted. This type is quite common in both Sjögren's syndrome and FM. Common causes of sleep disruption include joint or muscle pain and having to get up frequently to go to the bathroom due to a high level of fluid intake during the day in an effort to relieve dry mouth and throat.

Increasing Your Energy

◆ Listen to your body and rest when you need it. Some people find they really benefit from or even need a rest in bed in the early afternoon, and doing so allows them to get going again.

◆ Alternate rest with exercise. Gradually increasing your exercise may also help decrease your fatigue.

◆ Talk to your doctor about any medications that might contribute to fatigue, such as tranquilizers. However, be sure to continue to take any medications prescribed for Sjögren's syndrome unless your doctor feels they should be discontinued, and then follow carefully any directions for withdrawal. Never abruptly discontinue a medication without medical advice.

◆ Don't skip meals, especially breakfast. Bear in mind that improving your diet may increase your energy level.

◆ Reduce your use of caffeine, nicotine, sugary foods, and alcohol, which tend to contribute to fatigue.

◆ Cut back on watching television, and instead spend time with friends, try new activities, or travel to break the fatigue cycle.

◆ Bear in mind that tiredness may be related to another health problem, such as thyroid problems or depression. Consult your doctor if fatigue persists despite your best endeavors.

Getting a Good Night's Sleep

Whatever the reasons for poor sleep, it is important not to let them become ingrained. Here are some tips for establishing a good sleep pattern:

- Tackle the specific causes of sleep disruption. For example, excessive urination during the night can be remedied by sucking on ice chips during the day, using humidifiers, and applying oral lubricants or saliva substitutes.

- Stick to the same bedtime and try to get up at the same time each morning. Try not to oversleep no matter how poorly you have slept the night before.

- If you can't sleep, sit in bed and undertake a restful activity, such as reading, knitting, or doing a puzzle. Such activity takes the pressure off you to get to sleep.

- Ensure you have enough daily exercise, but avoid exercise in the evening, as it can leave you too stimulated to sleep.

- Try stress reduction techniques, such as meditation, biofeedback, or progressive relaxation.

- Avoid caffeine after lunch and alcohol after dinner, and consider eliminating them altogether. For some people, even one cup of coffee or one alcoholic drink is enough to disturb sleep.

- The bedroom should be quiet, dark, and comfortable. Don't use it for work. Try to create a restful association with sleep in this room.

- During the daytime, try to expose your body to at least one hour of natural light. Some evidence shows it can strengthen circadian rhythms and improve the quality of sleep.

Sometimes, following good sleep habits does not improve sleep or relieve daytime fatigue, in which case you should consult your doctor about possible specific sleep disorders. For example, sleep apnea is a condition in which breathing is interrupted during sleep. Snoring or gasping for breath upon waking can be signs of sleep apnea, a condition that can arise from the weight gain that often accompanies the use of corticosteroids. Diagnosis of any sleep disorder requires evaluation by a specialist and treatment, so your doctor may refer you to a sleep expert.

Making Your Bed Comfortable

Some people with Sjögren's find it helps to make minor changes to their bed, although it may not work for everyone. With this kind of illness, the focus needs to be on finding out what helps you as an individual. Even though it didn't work for Mandy in Chapter 1, a new mattress may indeed help someone else!

- ◆ Take the weight off painful feet and ankles by making a dome or a kind of tent toward the lower end of the bed to lift bedclothes off your lower limbs.

- ◆ Place a board beneath the mattress to provide extra support for your back, especially if you spend long periods of time in bed.

- ◆ Put a board laid across the bottom half of the mattress to enable you to exercise gently by walking your feet back and forth under the dome while lying down.

- ◆ Help circulation and relieve the joints from the pressure of gravity by using a slant board, which gently tilts your head down in the bed. If you suffer from reflux, you may prefer to raise the head of your bed by a few inches.

Not Forgetting Sex

At a time when Sjögren's syndrome may be attacking your lifestyle and identity, a loss of intimacy can be particularly upsetting. Some people feel too exhausted or unwell for much physical contact but may feel they're missing out emotionally. As time goes on, your relationship with your partner may become strained. The following are some suggestions on making physical contact more comfortable and enjoyable:

◆ Aim for effective pain control. Look at the advice in Chapter 6 on managing pain and consult your doctor about medication.

◆ Alleviate vaginal dryness with artificial lubricants, as described in Chapter 3.

◆ Don't underestimate tiredness as a cause of lost desire. Have a look at the suggestions for beating fatigue in this chapter.

◆ Eat as well as possible. Look at the section on diet in this chapter and also consider the advice on supplements in Chapter 5.

◆ Consult your doctor if you fear you may be anemic. Fatigue caused by anemia can kill all interest in close contact.

◆ Don't minimize the importance of a good cuddle if you don't feel up to sex!

Diet

A healthy diet is part of taking care of yourself under any circumstances and is doubly important if you have Sjögren's, although adopting one may require some thought and adjustment. A sore and dry mouth, possible gingivitis, and tooth problems may make a normal diet less appetizing; yet, now is the time when you need to obtain the maximum nutrients from your food.

Generally, you may find you get on better with moister, more fluid foods, such as soups, casseroles, mousses, smoothies, and the like. Such foods may take a little more preparation but are worth the extra effort if you are using fresh ingredients. A better diet will result in better health and improved energy levels.

Try to avoid alcoholic drinks and caffeine, which are dehydrating and can contribute to increased dryness. Spicy and acidic food can also irritate your mouth, and sugary food can promote tooth decay.

The lack of saliva has important implications. Any foods likely to erode tooth enamel should be avoided, such as sugary drinks, alcohol, and citrus fruits like lemons. Hot and spicy foods may also need to be cut out or limited, such as curries, foods containing chili, and some fast or packaged foods that can be hard on the moisture-producing glands.

Some people have found they react badly to a number of common food additives. Some Sjögren's symptoms may diminish if you avoid substances like monosodium glutamate (MSG), the artificial sweetener aspartame (Nutrasweet), and the preservative citric acid (which causes mouth sores in some).

A high intake of calcium (in dairy products, such as milk, cheese, and yogurt) will help boost tooth health. Plain live yogurt may also help prevent thrush in the mouth. Some people with Sjögren's develop lactose intolerance, so must turn to other good sources of calcium, such as dark green leafy vegetables, sesame seeds, canned fish (with the bones), hard water, dried figs, bread, and the humble baked bean!

Incorporating Essential Fatty Acids (EFAs)

Found in several fish and vegetable oils, EFAs play a vital role in good heart health and promote the smooth running of the immune and nervous systems. We need EFAs to manufacture and repair cell membranes and to produce prostaglandins. Prostaglandins regulate body functions such as heart rate, blood pressure, blood clotting, fertility, and conception and play a role in immune function by regulating inflammation and encouraging the body to fight infection. Lack of EFAs has been linked with several health conditions, including heart disease and cancer, as well as other autoimmune disorders, such as lupus and rheumatoid arthritis. There is some evidence that EFAs also help reduce inflammation. There are two types: omega-6 and omega-3.

Omega-6

Omega-6, or linolenic acid, is found in the following:

- Vegetables
- Fruits
- Nuts
- Grains
- Seeds
- Butter
- Oils made from evening primrose, pumpkin, and wheat germ

Omega-3

One tablespoon a day of flaxseed oil provides the recommended daily adult portion of omega-3. Also known as alpha-linoleic acid, there are many sources, including:

- Fish oil
- Butter
- Flaxseed (linseed)
- Mustard seed
- Pumpkin seed
- Soy bean
- Walnut oil
- Green leafy vegetables
- Grains
- Spirulina
- Oils made from linseed (flaxseed) or soy beans

How to Make the Best of EFAs

High heat, light, and oxygen destroy EFAs, so when consuming foods for their EFA content, try to avoid cooked or heated forms. For example, raw nuts are a better source than roasted nuts. Don't use flaxseed oil for cooking, and never reuse any type of oil. Extra virgin olive oil or grapeseed oil are best to use as cooking oil, as they withstand high heat well.

Replace hydrogenated fats (like margarine) and polyunsaturated fats (common cooking oils) with healthy EFA-based fats when possible. For example, instead of using margarine on your vegetables, use flaxseed and/or extra virgin olive oils.

Another idea is to grind flaxseed to sprinkle on vegetables for a slightly nutty taste. Whole flaxseeds are usually passed through the intestine, simply absorbing water and not yielding much oil.

Addressing Swallowing Problems

For those people with Sjögren's who have problems swallowing, it can be all too easy to limit your choice of foods to what is easiest or most convenient and end up with an inadequate diet. To maximize the benefits from your food choices, consider the following:

- Make the most of soups by using a blender. Meat, vegetables, lentils, soy beans, and other beans can all be puréed to make nourishing liquid meals.

- Add eggs, cheese, or tofu to increase protein.

- Make casseroles and cut food into bite-sized or smaller pieces (a pair of scissors is handy for meat) when making the sauce.

- Mash or purée vegetables and fruits.

- Make sauces more interesting by using yogurt, tomatoes, and low-fat fromage frais.

- Consider buying a juicer to make wonderful combinations

of vegetables (such as carrot and beet) or fruit (such as blueberry and banana).

♦ Make the most of eggs, which are nourishing and versatile. Try them scrambled, poached, or made into custards.

♦ Try Jell-O, ice creams, custards, milk shakes, and smoothies. Adding silken tofu to these will boost protein.

♦ Eat a number of small meals or snacks during the course of the day, rather than one or two big ones.

♦ Rinse your mouth regularly to remove debris, add freshness, and lubricate your mouth.

Digestive Problems

Julia found she had a lot of abdominal discomfort. Eating too much wheat and dairy products in particular seemed to upset her delicate digestive balance, resulting in gassy pains and bloating. She was never sure whether to connect this with her Sjögren's, with stress, or both.

Lack of moisture can affect the esophagus and other inner digestive organs. For example, some people with Sjögren's suffer from low intestinal mucous secretions, which can cause irritable bowel syndrome (IBS), constipation, lower abdominal pain, and alterations in bowel habits. To counter these potential problems, try increasing the amount of fiber in your diet.

Increase Fiber

♦ Use whole-grain breads and cereals as croutons in soup, as breadcrumbs to top casseroles or puddings, or as dumplings in casseroles.

♦ Try to eat apples and potatoes unpeeled.

♦ Make soups with dried beans or legumes.

- Add dates or figs to puddings or make into sauces to go with ice cream.

- Make raw soups sometimes, such as uncooked tomatoes and fresh parsley or carrot and orange juice.

- Try finely grated salads, such as carrot and raisin or red cabbage.

- Top salads with seeds, such as sunflower, sesame, or pumpkin seeds.

Eliminate Food Allergens

Food allergy or intolerance may be implicated in Sjögren's. Common foods that cause allergy or intolerance include milk products, eggs, nuts, fish and shellfish, wheat and flour, chocolate, artificial colors, pork and bacon, chicken, tomatoes, soft fruit, and yeast. The most common symptoms of allergy include asthma, gastrointestinal symptoms (nausea, vomiting, and diarrhea), eczema, urticaria (hives), rhinorrhea (heavy discharge from the nose), and angioedema (swelling of the blood vessels). Other more long-term symptoms can include depression, anxiety, fatigue, migraine, and sleeplessness.

Whether these symptoms result from diet or Sjögren's can be difficult to determine, but possible allergens can be detected with a scratch or blood test or an elimination diet. If you think that excluding or limiting a food will help improve your quality of life, it may be worth a try. Eliminate all suspected allergens for two weeks and reintroduce them one by one by eating one of the foods three times in one day. Watch for a reaction for three days before introducing another food.

Avoid Heartburn

Because saliva normally plays such a major role in neutralizing stomach acid, some people with Sjögren's find they are more prone to heartburn. Antacids may help. You can also try raising the head of your bed, using two or three books or wood blocks, to prevent gastric acid from washing back into the esophagus at night. If your problem is severe, discuss medication with your doctor. Bear in mind that medicines containing sucralfate, designed to coat the esophagus and stomach, might actually interfere with the absorption of other medications.

Take Coated Tablets

Because saliva normally helps you swallow things, you may find that pills—especially if large—can become stuck to dry walls of the esophagus, causing pain and sometimes a feeling of choking. This can have implications if you need to take medications at regular intervals but aren't digesting them on time because they are getting stuck halfway down.

Arrange to take coated tablets when possible. Take medication with plenty of water, while sitting or standing, and don't lie down immediately afterward.

Smoking

This one is easy—don't do it! Apart from its more widely publicized health effects, smoking is exceedingly drying and can damage your mouth, nose, eyes, and lungs, making symptoms of Sjögren's worse. In fact, few people with Sjögren's are smokers, and this may be a silver lining of the disease!

If you have not yet stopped, here are some suggestions to help you on your way:

- Prepare yourself for quitting; set a special day, such as a birthday or anniversary.

- Read as much information on stopping smoking as you can.

- Involve a friend and get someone to stop smoking with you (if possible).

◆ Be realistic. You will have withdrawal symptoms, but they will go away.

◆ Keep a diary and note when you tend to smoke and what triggers the need to light up. Then try and avoid those situations.

◆ Calculate how much money you'll save by not smoking— and plan what you could spend the money on.

◆ Take magnesium to help reduce cravings.

◆ If you do relapse, be positive and consider it a learning experience. Just go back to your quitting plan. Most people have a few goes at it before they finally stop smoking.

Travel

There is no reason why you shouldn't travel, provided you pace yourself so it doesn't become too tiring. Listed below are a few hints that hopefully will make your journey more enjoyable.

◆ *Medication.* Take enough of each of your medications to last you through the entire trip. In fact, a spare set can be useful in case one gets lost. Put one set in your hand luggage and pack the other in your suitcase.

◆ *Time zones.* If you're changing time zones and are on medication, ask your doctor's advice about whether this will affect your medication.

◆ *Air travel.* Notoriously drying, airplanes can present special challenges to those with Sjögren's. Stay hydrated by moistening your nasal passages with a saline solution and drinking plenty of water at regular intervals. If you feel unwell while flying, tell a flight attendant. They are well trained and equipped for emergencies.

◆ *Travel sickness pills.* Be careful about taking these, as they may exacerbate mouth dryness.

- *Luggage.* Most of us take far too much! A good general rule is to take half the amount of clothes you think you will need. The last thing you want is to exhaust yourself dragging around a heavy case. Use lightweight bags, wheeled cases, or trolleys, and/or hire a porter or skycap.

Stress

Stress definitely makes Sjögren's worse for some people. Patricia, a young mother of two, made her own list of personal de-stressors after realizing there was a direct link between how much stress she experienced and how bad her condition was. Her list included:

- Make no major decisions.

- Stop rushing and pace myself.

- Check what food I've been eating and eat some fresh fruit if I've eaten a lot of junk food.

- Get some sunlight or daylight.

- Change my routine.

- Play with the children.

- Talk to someone.

- Modify my expectations so they are more realistic.

- Write down three positive statements about my life.

Richard, a rare male with Sjögren's who also suffers from lupus, says he drops everything and gets out of the house or office as soon as possible if he's feeling stressed. "Of course, it's not always possible if I'm in a meeting, but just planning to get away for a few minutes is a big help. It gives me a feeling of control and I know that once out in the open air I forget my frustration very quickly."

It may help to make a list of the things that cause stress in your life and how these affect you, your family, and your job. Questions to ask yourself could be:

- Is the stress short- or long-term?

- How much control do I have over it or do I perceive someone else to be in charge (i.e., boss, partner) of my life. If I am not in control, up to what point can I accept this?

- What are my biggest obstacles to reducing stress?

- Do I have a support system of friends and/or family that will help me make positive changes?

- What am I willing to change or give up for a less stressful and tension-filled life?

Tips for Reducing or Controlling Stress

Beating stress may take time and determination, especially if it has persisted for a while. If your stress level is really severe you may need to consider lifestyle changes. Chronic stress can sometimes be a wake-up call summoning you to a change of job, a change of career, or other major shifts in your life. We all have an individual tolerance level for stress, so, as with other aspects of Sjögren's, it is a matter of finding your own limits and doing your best to live within these limits, rather than just paying lip service to them.

There is nothing noble about enduring stressful situations, so try to change or avoid them. If they are unavoidable, such as getting through a long working day, work out a compromise. Take short breaks or go somewhere quiet for a few minutes. If you can, take a hot bath or sit quietly and listen to soothing music. Take time to unwind and gather your resources. If preserving your health means you must negotiate with an employer, do it with the confidence that comes from knowing that compromise is a constructive solution.

- *Learn how to pace yourself.* Adapt a moderate pace, keep a regular schedule, and get adequate rest and exercise.

- *Learn to say no.* This is perhaps the most important stress-management skill you can master, and it's especially important to pace yourself on days when you feel energetic and may be tempted to overdo it.

♦ *Wait before making a decision.* Bear in mind that you can make a more well-informed decision after further consideration. If you're not sure whether to say yes or no to an activity, a useful phrase is, "May I come back to you on that one?" Points to consider include: Can I realistically do this? Is it better to say no at the start, rather than embroil myself and then find I don't have the strength to finish? How much can I do? Is the deadline realistic? What adjustments can I make?

♦ *Don't hesitate to ask for help if you need it.* You can ask for help with chores or ask for a sympathetic ear. But if you think that you may be under more stress than just a passing difficulty, it may be helpful to talk with your doctor, who may be able to suggest professional counseling.

♦ *Assess your responsibilities.* Are you taking on more than you can or should handle?

♦ *Be realistic, not perfect.* You may expect too much of yourself and others, and then feel frustrated or let down when matters turn out less than perfectly.

♦ *Go easy with criticism of others and yourself.* Try suspending all judgments for a day. Give in occasionally, even if you think you're in the right. Put your health and peace of mind first.

♦ *Meditate.* Just ten to twenty minutes of quiet reflection may bring relief from chronic stress as well as increase your tolerance to it. Use the time to listen to music, relax, and try to think of pleasant things or nothing.

♦ *Visualize.* Use your imagination and picture how you can manage a stressful situation more successfully. Whether it's a business presentation or moving to a new place, many people feel visual rehearsals boost self-confidence and enable them to take a more positive approach to a difficult task.

◆ *Break down tasks.* Do one task at a time. When you're stressed, even a normal workload can sometimes feel overwhelming, so try to tackle one part of your job at a time. If you feel very stressed, start with something very simple, such as putting a letter in an envelope. As trivial as it sounds, performing any activity, regardless of how minor, can help you break down the feeling that you can't cope.

◆ *Exercise.* Regular exercise is a popular way to relieve stress. Twenty to thirty minutes of physical activity two or three times a week benefits both the body and the mind.

◆ *Keep up hobbies.* Take a break from your worries by doing something you enjoy. Whether it's gardening or painting, schedule time to indulge in your interest.

◆ *Adopt a healthy lifestyle.* Good nutrition makes a difference, and you should minimize your intake of caffeine and alcohol or cut them out entirely. Get enough rest, and balance exercise, work, and relaxation.

Relaxation and Creative Visualization

These techniques may take some practice, but they work together, not just to ease tension but to promote a more positive outlook and self-image. You can, of course, choose the images that suit you best, but a sample relaxation scenario can be as follows:

Imagine you are setting off from home. You enter a beautiful forest with a cool, clear stream running through it. There are fish swimming in the stream. You climb up a gentle slope and find a bench, where you sit for a while. You think of all the things that are worrying or hurting you, one by one, and give each one a color and a shape. When you get up from the bench, you leave these "objects" behind you and walk away from them.

You keep walking through the forest until at last it opens out onto a beautiful sandy cove. The sea is washing gently onto the shore and birds are calling overhead. The sun is warm but not too hot or bright.

You find a comfortable spot and sit down, leaning back against the warm cliff-face and closing your eyes as you listen to the swish of the sea and the cries of the birds. You feel calm, untroubled, serene.

You stay there for a while and then, as afternoon draws near, you decide it is time to leave. You open your eyes, stand up, and return home, knowing that you can come back to this place any time you close your eyes, and that when you do you will feel the same calmness again.

Chapter 8

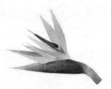

Exercise and Physiotherapy

It's generally agreed that mild exercise can be beneficial for those with Sjögren's syndrome. Gentle activities, such as walking or swimming, can help keep joints and muscles flexible, and may also boost your energy and mood, as well as protect against further joint damage. However, there may well be times when you feel just too exhausted to manage anything. The trick is to balance rest and activity.

To Rest or Not to Rest?

For many people, the pain and stiffness associated with Sjögren's are often worse first thing in the morning, and the temptation is probably to do as little as possible. The same temptation probably applies at other times during the day, especially if you suffer from so-called inflammatory fatigue, also known as late-morning or early-afternoon fatigue, when you may get up feeling vigorous but find your energy suddenly evaporates later on in the day.

Rest is certainly a vital part of coping with Sjögren's, and it is important to listen to your body and not to push yourself too far. Don't feel guilty about taking the rest you need, especially if you have fever and fatigue. Regular rest periods can be key in helping you to pace yourself.

At the same time, it's also generally recognized that it is better for your overall physical health—and mental well-being—if you partake in regular, mild exercise. In the olden days, some thirty or forty years ago, people were sometimes taken into a hospital and given bed rest for weeks or months to help soothe inflamed joints—sometimes with their limbs in splints. With too much bed rest, unused muscles become weaker, bones lose calcium and become more brittle, and your general physical fitness level declines.

Times have changed, and your doctor is now more likely to advise a nice walk or gentle swim! The balance of rest and exercise can be a fine one, but both need to be maintained with Sjögren's.

Exercise has several important functions in Sjögren's syndrome. One of the most important functions is to maintain and maximize the mobility of any affected joints. Regular aerobic exercise builds up the resilience and capacity of the heart, lungs, and circulation.

Research at the University of Missouri found that strengthening exercises and low-impact aerobic exercise for people with arthritis resulted in improved stamina, less fatigue, and an improved level of general physical functioning. As stiff and painful joints are symptoms of both arthritis and Sjögren's, the results can be taken as encouraging for people who suffer from either or both disorders.

Exercise improves quality of life, resulting in less muscle tension, lower stress and anxiety levels, improved energy levels, increased self-esteem, and a better night's sleep. It also helps to strengthen bones and guards against osteoporosis.

Laura was the world's worst exerciser—until she started getting short of breath. She would puff and pant by the time she got to the top of the stairs and was thoroughly frightened that she had heart disease, asthma, or some unknown complication of her Sjögren's. She felt she must have more fresh air and started taking daily walks outside. This simple measure improved her fitness and well-being beyond what she could have imagined. She now manages a swim once a week or once every two weeks. It's still not enough, she feels, but it's better than nothing and a lot better than before.

Which Exercise?

Individual exercise programs vary greatly. Laura was keen on her daily walk, Julia was a yoga devotee, and Kimberley worked with a physiotherapist from the hospital rheumatology department on exercises designed to help her painful joints.

In general, short and frequent exercise sessions are better than long bouts of exercise. Alternating exercise and rest is also recommended. Look for ways to possibly combine the two, such as lying down while doing a gentle exercise like rotating the ankles and wrists, for example.

There are different types of exercises:

◆ *Range-of-motion exercises* reduce stiffness and help keep your joints moving. A range-of-motion exercise for your shoulder would mean moving your arm in a large circle.

◆ *Moderate stretching exercises* help relieve the pain and keep the muscles and tendons around an affected joint flexible and strong.

◆ *Strengthening exercises* maintain or increase muscle strength.

◆ *Endurance exercises* strengthen your heart, give you energy, and keep your body flexible. These exercises include walking, swimming, and cycling.

Range-of-Motion and Moderate Stretching Exercises

Range-of-motion exercises are important for those with Sjögren's, especially when the joints are inflamed during a flare-up. The goal is to reduce stiffness and minimize loss of mobility in the affected joints. This type of exercise takes the joint through the fullest range of movement that it can manage once or twice a day or whenever you feel the need to reduce stiffness. Pay special attention to the point at which movement becomes difficult or impossible and don't push the joint to the point of pain. Once the acute inflammation has died down, range-of-motion exercises become part of the warm-up to the daily exercise routine, which commonly includes a ten-minute warm-up, a fifteen-minute workout, and a five-minute cool-down.

Stretching is a variation on range-of-motion exercise. It involves stretching the joint to just beyond the limit of comfort, as opposed to staying just within the comfort zone. No one will tell you to stretch to the level of actual pain, and you shouldn't bounce the joint in an attempt to extend it further. By putting the joint through its paces regularly, stiffness and pain are reduced. Range-of-motion exercises are even better done in water because the buoyancy of the water supports the body and protects the joints from rapid or stressful movement.

Strengthening Exercises

Muscles that may have become weak through lack of use need to be rebuilt gradually through exercise. Strengthening exercises come at different levels. For example, isotonic exercises involve contracting the muscle and moving the joint by, for example, lifting weights.

In contrast, isometric strengthening exercises involve clenching and unclenching muscle groups without external movement. These exercises can be done lying or sitting down, and they work by introducing an external pressure point. For example, you might push against a sofa, tightening your arm muscles without moving wrists, elbows, or shoulders. Such exercises should be part of your routine, even when the joints are seriously inflamed, in order to minimize the weakening of muscles from disuse, and can probably be used after a flare-up when inflammation has died down. Don't try push-ups, however, as they can be too much of a strain.

Endurance Exercises

Just as your leg and arm muscles become weak with disuse, so do the heart, lungs, and blood vessels if not made to work. Cardiovascular exercise ("cardio" for heart, "vascular" refers to the blood vessels, and lung function is also involved) is important for general fitness. Such exercise increases the capacity of the heart, lungs, and blood vessels to work efficiently under stress by using oxygen efficiently.

The best kind of cardiovascular exercise for someone with Sjögren's will involve moderate effort but no jolting of joints (as in impact exercise). Instead, try swimming (the breaststroke rather than crawl if the shoulders are affected), walking, cycling, and climbing up and down stairs (unless the knees are inflamed).

Depending on the joints affected, some form of low-impact aerobic exercise—like bouncing a ball or dancing (the waltz, not salsa)—may also be attempted once the inflammation is in retreat. When the muscles show signs of regaining strength and supporting affected joints adequately, it may be possible to start working with weights, under professional guidance.

Don't Overdo It

You may have heard exercise fanatics talk about "feeling the burn." However, "no pain, no gain" does not apply here! It's probably good if you aim to be a little bit breathless after exercise, because it shows that the activity has increased your heart rate and so improved your cardiovascular performance and stamina. However, take heed of any warning signs, such as pain, shortness of breath, prolonged fatigue, dizziness, chest pain, or increased joint pain—and stop. Don't push your body.

Build up a routine gradually. Start with just five minutes at a time or with three or four gentle stretches or yoga positions. Then try building up to ten to fifteen minutes three times a day and increasing this to half an hour of exercise several times a week.

Remember you are doing this to keep as fit and healthy as possible, not to compete as a professional athlete. If you find yourself suffering, stop.

How to Get the Best from Your Exercise

Walking, swimming, and cycling are three excellent ways to get the exercise you need. Depending on your state of health and circumstances, you'll probably find that one suits you better than the others. For example, if you suffer from painful leg joints or extreme fatigue, you may prefer cycling or swimming to walking.

Walking

- Warm up for walking by doing range-of-motion exercises for knees and hips.

- Soak your feet in warm water and do range-of-motion foot exercises.

- Wear supportive walking shoes or athletic sneakers with good shock absorbers.

- Walk on a flat surface whenever possible (beside a river); avoid hills.

- Swing your arms for balance while walking.

- Soak feet in cool water if they feel warm after a walk.

Cycling

- Adjust the seat height of your saddle so that your legs are fully straightened when pedalling.

- Set the handlebars so that they are not too low or far away from the saddle. A prone position puts strain on the lower back, shoulders, elbows, and wrists.

- Adjust the pedal tension to the lowest level to limit strain on the knees.

- Ride an indoor exercise bike if the weather is bad.

- Use an indoor bike with arm motion attachments if you start feeling pain in your knees.

- Cool down with light pedalling as a substitute for range-of-motion exercises.

Swimming

- Do a training session under the guidance of a trained physiotherapist, if possible.

- Breathe regularly from your diaphragm during exercise.

- Check the temperature of the pool before swimming. Temperatures between 82°F and 86°F are best for aerobic exercise. Higher temperatures than this increase vaso-dilatation (expansion of blood vessels) and may make you feel light headed. Temperatures up to 92°F or 98°F are suitable for range-of-motion and stretching exercise but not for serious swimming.

- Don't go swimming with a fever or an open wound, or if you have a history of uncontrolled seizures or either high or low blood pressure.

Heat

Heat reduces pain and soothes and relaxes the mind and body. It works by causing the blood vessels to expand, increasing the blood flow to the area and generally speeding up the metabolism.

Heat is especially useful as a prelude to exercise because joints perform better when warmed up. There are a number of different devices for delivering heat, most related to the domestic bath and hot-water bottle. There are whirlpool baths, infra-red heat lamps, hot packs, and electric heating pads. Heat application can be used in conjunction with gentle range-of-motion exercises as part of your exercise warm-up.

What you use depends on your preference, but bear in mind it is important not to overdo heat. Some people have the mistaken idea that hotter is better. It's not. If the skin begins to blotch, the heat is too great, and no matter how relaxing it is, you should never fall asleep while using heat treatment.

The use of cold is favored by some physiotherapists, and although it does not have the relaxing, psychological benefits associated with heat, in the case of seriously inflamed and swollen joints, the benefit of a cold application may be greater than that of heat.

Don't Forget to Warm Down

Sports experts emphasize the importance of warming down or cooling down after vigorous exercise to help reduce cramps and soreness in tired muscles. It also makes you more flexible and helps prevent injury. The idea is not to get cold, but to cool down gently. So when you do exercise vigorously, allow a few minutes at the end of the session to warm down with lighter exercise and stretching. A therapeutic massage also helps and is wonderfully relaxing.

Chapter 9

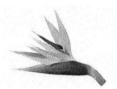

Coping With Your Feelings

Living with a condition such as Sjögren's involves uncertainty, which in turn can cause stress. Each person may have a different constellation of symptoms, sometimes from day to day, as *Laura* explains:

> Every day is different. One day I wake up feeling fine, the next I may be debilitated by poor sight, itchy skin, and aching limbs. My Sjögren's is certainly a mover and a shaker! It started with very itchy skin and then a red, swollen eye. My optician sent me off for arthritis tests, and meanwhile I developed a lump beneath my parotid gland at the side of my face. It's gone on from there, and frankly by now I don't know what to expect next. I can live a normal life—just about—but I'm always on the lookout for the next symptom.

People react in different ways to being diagnosed with Sjögren's. Emotions range from grief and depression to relief.

Grief

Mandy was happily married and had a career as a midwife, which she loved. Because she used her hands in her work a great deal, she took no notice at first when the last three fingers of her left hand were constantly sore. After some time, a colleague at work persuaded her to see her own family doctor, and after blood tests she was told she had rheumatoid arthritis. She was then referred to a rheumatologist for further treatment. Her condition worsened as the pain moved into both hands, wrists, elbows, knees, and ankles. She began to feel extremely tired, more so than the usual fatigue after shift work. She was always run down and caught every cold and flu that went around. She took long-term sick leave and was planning to give up the career she loved. On the advice of another doctor at the hospital where she worked, she saw a different rheumatologist, who immediately diagnosed Sjögren's. For Mandy, the diagnosis meant grief, as it threatened her job and meant the end of a certain personality she felt she had—happy and coping. In the end she took sick leave for nine months and then resumed on a part-time basis, which gave her a better balance of work and leisure.

Relief

Kimberley

I was so relieved to get a diagnosis because I can finally put a name to the never-ending series of health problems I've suffered from over the past five years. It is so good to know that it's not just all in my head and I'm *not* a hypochondriac.

Anger

Laura

I literally cry with anger. I feel that my illness contributed to the breakup of my most recent relationship and, frankly, I sometimes despair that I will never be able to have a long-term sexual relationship. I feel as if I'm one hundred years old and I'm only twenty-three. I feel this illness is cheating me out of my life.

Delayed Reaction

Christine

For a few years I dealt really well with the fact that I had a chronic condition, and I managed to lead a relatively normal life by working around my symptoms—I was so used to them, and I suppose I assumed they'd never worsen. Then life threw a few situations at me. First we relocated offices, which vastly added to my daily traveling, and then I was made redundant and didn't work for nearly a year. Then I had a miscarriage. Finally my father died unexpectedly. He was only fifty-seven. I think the combined stress of these life events influenced me. I certainly spiralled downhill over a period of about two years. Today I am learning to pace myself and take life much easier. I now have a local, part-time job, but the exhaustion and aches and pains are much worse. I seem to have chronic sinus problems, and my face keeps swelling up when I get overtired. I can only hope things get better and that I get back on the relatively even keel I was on previously.

Restoring a sense of control starts with gaining an understanding of your illness. Reading this book is an excellent start! What you know about your condition can make a difference in how you approach each day. So aim to be as well informed as possible. Ask your family doctor or specialist for information or find a support group through the Sjögren's Syndrome Foundation (see Resources).

Another useful information tool for you and your doctor is a medical diary. In it, keep track of your visits to the doctor—when and why. In addition, maintain a list of treatments and medications and any side effects. You may also want to include copies of your test results, as well as a record of symptoms, their severity, and possible triggers.

Emotional Ups and Downs

Living with a chronic illness can involve a roller coaster of emotions. There are several ways you can help even out the ups and downs:

- ◆ *Keep in touch.* Don't shut yourself away from the world, and do make the most of family and friends. A friend can help you break through negative feelings and suggest alternative ways of thinking, feeling, and behaving. Try to be with people even if you don't feel like talking. In particular, doing something for someone else boosts your self-esteem, helps you feel like a real person again, and offers relief from worries about what may happen to you.

♦ *Keep up ordinary everyday activities.* Stay involved, whether it's by going to concerts, singing in the church choir, or just meeting friends for lunch. Doing things you are used to or things you are good at establishes continuity that counteracts any feelings of disruption and loss.

♦ *Give yourself rewards.* Make a list of things you enjoy, such as favorite videos, pieces of music, favorite foods, places in the country, the seaside, or pets, and reward yourself by enjoying these things.

♦ *Find out as much as you can about your condition.* Learn your physical limits and the effects of the illness, as well as how to deal with any treatments, about Sjögren's syndrome in general, and your own state of health in particular. Strive for good communication with your doctors.

♦ *Talk to someone.* Most of the unpleasant emotions that plague people with a chronic illness are better out than in. By acknowledging and talking about feelings you gain more insight into them and are more able to change them for the better. You probably already have family, friends, or colleagues with whom you discuss your life, but it can be helpful to find people who also suffer from Sjögren's (see Resources).

Dealing With Depression

Depression is one of the most common complications of an ongoing or chronic illness like Sjögren's. This is natural. Not only are there the physical effects of the illness, there are psychological reactions as well. There may be loss of mobility and independence to contend with, and having a diagnosis of Sjögren's can change the way you see yourself and how you relate to others. In fact, it may require an in-depth reevaluation of your whole self-image.

It's worth bearing in mind that depression can often make pain and fatigue worse, thus aggravating the symptoms of Sjögren's. It can also increase any feelings of social isolation.

It is, however, quite possible to overlook the symptoms of depression, assuming that feeling depressed is normal for someone struggling with a serious, chronic illness. Symptoms of depression include the following:

♦ Feeling sad or depressed, with loss of interest or pleasure in daily activities

♦ Significant weight loss or weight gain

♦ Sleep disturbances, either sleeping too much or not being able to sleep

♦ Problems with concentration

♦ Apathy

♦ Feelings of worthlessness or guilt

♦ Fatigue or loss of energy

♦ Recurrent thoughts of death or suicide

Just as with Sjögren's itself, early diagnosis and treatment for depression are essential. People who get treatment for depression that occurs at the same time as a chronic disease often experience an improvement in their overall medical condition and a better quality of life, and they are more easily able to stick to their treatment plans.

Many antidepressant medicines are available to treat depression and can start to work within a few weeks, and more than 80 percent of people with depression can be treated successfully with medicine, psychotherapy, or a combination of both. These drugs work by altering the level of certain chemicals in the brain, which are responsible for transferring messages between brain cells.

Psychotherapy refers to a variety of techniques used to treat depression. It involves talking to a licensed professional who helps the depressed person understand his or her depression better and regain a sense of control and pleasure in life. One of the advantages of talking to professionals—not necessarily doctors, but those experienced in assessing psychological problems—is that they are able to judge whether your depression or anxiety is serious enough to be treated with drugs. Your doctor can refer you to a counselor, or you can contact a support organization (see Resources).

Dealing With Anger and Resentment

Not everyone with a diagnosis of Sjögren's will feel angry, but some people do. Perhaps you may be feeling, "Why me? What did I do to deserve this? Why is life so unfair?" Again, this is a natural reaction, and it is extremely helpful to acknowledge it.

It is quite natural to look for something or someone to blame when bad things happen to you. Some people may take it out on their doctors because they seem slow and uncaring; others may blame employers or work colleagues for not understanding their problems; still others may get annoyed with their family for not helping enough with domestic tasks or because they start to treat you like an invalid, which makes you feel like one.

- *Discharge the anger.* Talk to either to a close friend or to a therapist or e-mail others in an on-line support group (see Resources).

- *Channel some of your anger.* Anger is energy, so use it to try to solve the situations that are making you so cross. For example, you may need to discuss work issues with an employer or colleagues in a more assertive way, or you may need to be more assertive with your family and to set limits with them if necessary.

- *Scale down your expectations.* You are now someone coping with a chronic disease, which leaves less room for some things or means that some things take longer. One way to create more realistic expectations is to scale jobs down into small tasks. Rather than declare that you must clean the whole house, decide to focus on the bathroom or one other area instead. Only do the larger task when the smaller one becomes easy. And if and when you manage to build upon what you undertake, don't forget to congratulate yourself!

Managing Feelings with Your Partner and Family

It is natural to feel anger, sadness, and frustration, and your partner or other family members may also go through the same emotions. A chronic illness affects not only you, but also your children, partner, and parents. How do you rearrange your role from being someone who supports everyone else to being someone who needs support?

The first thing to do is to dismiss guilt. Tell yourself firmly that you have nothing to feel guilty about. No one is to blame for you getting Sjögren's—least of all you. The situation has to be dealt with, by you and by everyone involved with you. People who value your relationship will not mind making adjustments.

If you are the sort of person whom others rely on, much of your self-esteem may depend on that role. Sjögren's requires that you gain self-esteem in other ways. Just as it may have given you satisfaction to be needed, you can give others a chance to derive that sense of satisfaction by being responsible and caring toward you. It can be an act of generosity to allow others to give to you.

Both you and your partner may find it helpful to consider the following suggestions:

◆ Accept your feelings. Don't berate yourself if you are sad or resentful. These feelings are normal as you adjust to the changes that follow the diagnosis of a chronic illness.

◆ Communicate your feelings with your partner. Share your fears and frustrations in an honest but caring way.

♦ Include your family in the process of dealing with the diagnosis and its aftermath. Share information with any children in an age-appropriate way and give them a chance to share their own fears and resentments, too. Sometimes children blame themselves for what has happened, and it is important for them to air these and similar feelings. Whatever their age, they will cope much better if they have some understanding of what is going on.

♦ Explain to children any changes that will need to be made to their routine, such as someone else picking them up from school sometimes.

♦ Establish a support network outside the immediate family that is separate from the one your partner has so you each have a way of sharing private feelings about the chronic illness.

♦ Get professional help if necessary. When adjusting to chronic illness, it may be helpful to seek the guidance of a professional counselor to help each member of the family cope with the necessary changes in their own way.

♦ Use a teamwork approach. Work together to create a realistic plan for how to handle the children, housework, scheduling, and social calendar. As partners, recognize the limitations of the illness and set realistic expectations and goals—what must be done, what should be done, what might be done. Don't forget to plan for fun times that allow you to stay close and connected.

How to Help

Living with someone who has Sjögren's can be frightening and depressing, but there is much that partners, family, and friends can do to help. (Because most people with Sjögren's are women, "she" will be used here.)

- Do your best to be supportive, give encouragement, and offer hope. Be patient and understanding. Your help at this time is absolutely invaluable. Most importantly for you, be prepared to seek help, both for her and for yourself, if you feel you need it.

- Ask her what she needs and how best you can help. It may be that she has a clear idea of what help is needed. Perhaps you can take over the shopping for the week, ferry the children to school, act as a mediator between her and her doctor, or just sit and listen while she talks.

- Encourage her to accept help from others and to seek it from her doctor. Offer to accompany her to appointments if you think it may help.

- Suggest she join a support group (see Resources). Exchanging experiences with people in a similar position and realizing that you really are not the only one suffering can be an enormous relief. This may not be something she will feel she wants to do at first, but as she begins to feel better, she may change her mind. If it is appropriate, you could offer to go with her.

- Offer help with practical arrangements, such as child care, cleaning, washing, ironing, and so on.

- Be patient. Remember that Sjögren's is an illness. She cannot help suffering the symptoms that she does. Hopefully she is doing all she can to make herself think positively and feel better.

- Let her express her true feelings, even if it is not easy for you to hear what she has to say. You may feel that you are hearing the same things again and again, and wonder if talking is really helping her. Some people need to talk about something endlessly; some people may not want to talk about it very much at all. Whatever suits the person is to be encouraged.

♦ Find out as much as you can about Sjögren's syndrome, especially if she is frightened of what she may find out or just feels too ill to study the condition herself.

♦ Give her treats—a cuddle, a cup of tea in bed, a special phone call or text message.

♦ Ensure that she gets enough food and rest. Leave a prepared meal for her in the fridge the evening before.

♦ Encourage her to be active. Consider going for a short walk together on a regular basis.

♦ Give her a massage. You don't need to be an expert; most of us aren't! Try some gentle stroking of her neck, shoulders, and back to start. If you and she prefer, massage her feet.

♦ Get help if you need it. Don't keep your problems to yourselves. Talk to your doctor or seek help from organizations that offer advice and support (see Resources).

♦ Last but not least, try not to slip into the age-old temptation of telling her to pull herself together. She will not appreciate it. If she could, she would—even though she may be applying the same advice to herself! Instead, reassure her of your love and support.

Positive Thinking

There is some confusion about positive thinking and illness—a kind of uneasy feeling that if you think positive thoughts hard enough, you ought to be able to magically banish the Sjögren's from your body. Conversely, if the condition persists, it may seem as if it is your fault because you are not positive enough. Some people may fear that feeling sad or having negative feelings will delay their recovery or make the Sjögren's worse.

You may also be told by other people to think positively if you feel low or tearful, or want to talk about the hard fact that you have a chronic illness for which there is no known cure.

Such remarks from others can add to any feelings of confusion you are already feeling.

Being positive does not mean curing or banishing your Sjögren's, and it is not your fault if your illness persists! Being positive also does not mean you have to feel happy and cheerful all of the time. It is actually positive to acknowledge when you feel sad, tired, or angry. You are allowed to state when you are finding life difficult or just to have a good cry when it all gets too much. Tears are a natural response to distress and can be a healthy release for you.

Positive thinking means different things to different people, but generally it is about facing up to the Sjögren's. People do this in different ways. Some take a more active part in their treatment, reading all they can, surfing the Internet, and talking to lots of people. Others prefer to leave matters more in the hands of their doctors. Still others prefer to ignore the whole thing and just carry on as normally as possible.

Bear in mind that it is easier to feel positive if you are eating and sleeping well and getting enough rest and exercise. You may also find it helpful to deal with any underlying psychological or emotional issues that may be gnawing away at your sense of well-being.

That said, when you focus your attention on positive thoughts, ideas, and images, you tend to feel better. The link between a positive attitude and good health is well documented. One study of psychosomatic medicine found that people with a positive attitude were less likely to catch colds than those who were depressed, nervous, or angry. The study also found that uptight or sad people are more likely to complain of cold symptoms, even when they don't have a cold.

How to Be More Positive

♦ *On a daily basis, make a list of ten things you have accomplished.* Don't overlook small things, such as choosing a nice outfit for the day, tidying a room, or calling a friend.

- *Choose an accomplishment symbol.* This symbol is a task you normally do each day that you endow with the power to represent an accomplishment. Your accomplishment symbol may be brushing your teeth, washing your face, shaving, or having breakfast. Remember, it is something you are already doing, not something you think you should be doing. Whenever you do this task, you can enjoy a sense of accomplishment.

- *Interpret events differently.* Find a positive interpretation to the negatives in your life. If a negative thought comes to you, turn it around so the focus shifts from what you have lost to what you still have.

- *Exercise.* It's well known that exercise gives you a natural high by releasing natural body chemicals—endorphins—which reduce pain and lift the spirits. Exercise also concentrates the mind because it involves effort and gives you less opportunity to indulge in unpleasant thoughts.

Chapter 10

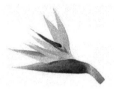

Becoming a Parent

What if you have Sjögren's and are planning to become pregnant? Or what if you are already a parent and have just been diagnosed? It is very easy to be afraid of not being able to cope when you are in pain or facing your very first pregnancy, but with information, support, and planning, you can find ways to be a happy and fulfilled parent who has Sjögren's.

The main point is to inform your doctor if you are planning to become pregnant. Most pregnancies are straightforward, but in a very few cases you might need extra tests for certain rare conditions, described more fully below. If possible, ask to be referred to an obstetrician who is knowledgeable about Sjögren's and make sure you have any necessary tests and treatments to optimize your chances of having a healthy baby.

Miscarriage

It is important to remember that miscarriage is common and can happen very easily even in cases where a woman is totally healthy. According to the National Center for Health Statistics, in 1996, miscarriage affected about 16.5 percent of women who became pregnant, and it is generally thought that between 15 and 20 percent of pregnancies end in miscarriage in the first trimester or early in the second trimester. Whatever the cause—and often it is impossible to determine—women generally find it deeply distressing to lose a baby in this way. Lack of support and information can exacerbate the distress, so if you have suffered miscarriage, ask your practitioner about local support groups or contact an on-line support group such as the International Council on Infertility Dissemination (see Resources).

Some women report recurrent miscarriages that they feel are linked to Sjögren's syndrome. While research on this is not extensive, a few women with Sjögren's may have antiphospholipid antibodies, sometimes called anticardiolipin antibodies, which can be associated with recurrent miscarriages, especially during the second trimester of pregnancy. These antibodies may cause clots to form in the placenta, interrupting the flow of blood to the fetus. Fortunately, you can be tested for these, and medication is available in the form of aspirin, heparin, or prednisolone. This condition is called antiphospholipid syndrome (APS) and is commonly, but not always, associated with lupus. For more information on APS, I recommend Triona Holden's book on the subject, *Positive Options for Antiphospholipid Syndrome* (Hunter House Publishers, 2003).

Can the Baby Inherit Sjögren's?

There is no proven hereditary link, although it is possible that a genetic tendency to Sjögren's may be passed on. However, experts believe that a trigger is still needed to turn it into an active syndrome. Research into this aspect of Sjögren's is being conducted in the United States and in Europe. So this should not be something you spend time worrying about, although you may want to discuss it with your doctor if you do have concerns.

Pregnancy

In the vast majority of cases, pregnancy is straightforward. On rare occasions, however, in pregnant women with Sjögren's syndrome who also have antibodies to Ro and La, the antibodies cross the placenta and affect the baby, resulting in a condition called neonatal lupus.

In the vast majority of cases this condition is not serious and does not need treatment, as it usually disappears within a few weeks. Neonatal lupus is not to be confused with lupus (systemic lupus erythematosus) and doesn't develop into it.

In its mild and most common form, neonatal lupus may take the form of a rash on the face and head or scattered over the body. This tends to appear a few days or weeks after birth, particularly after sun exposure, and usually disappears after a few more weeks as the mother's antibodies are slowly metabolized by the baby. As the rash looks much like any other baby rash, it can be identified by doing a blood test.

Another effect of neonatal lupus is a low blood count, perhaps resulting in anemia. Again, this effect is seldom serious and usually resolves without treatment in a few weeks. Liver disease is another effect that also usually clears up soon after birth.

Much more rarely, the baby's heart may be affected, resulting in a heart rhythm abnormality known as congenital heart block. This is a disorder in which the electrical signal that regulates the unborn baby's heartbeat is disrupted by abnormal antibodies. As a result, the heartbeat becomes very slow. Even in mothers with the Ro antibody, this complication occurs in fewer than one in one hundred pregnancies.

A normal heartbeat starts in the upper heart (the atria or auricles) and travels smoothly through to the bottom of the heart (the ventricles). In heart block, the atrial beat (about 140 times per minute in a newborn) cannot get through to the ventricles because scar tissue blocks its path. The ventricles then have to beat on their own (about sixty times per minute in a newborn). As the ventricle beat determines the pulse, the baby has an abnormally slow pulse.

The baby's pulse can be detected on scans from about twelve to fifteen weeks of pregnancy. If the unborn baby has a heart block but appears to be doing well—which is usually the case—either nothing is done or a special form of cortisone is given that will travel through the placenta to the baby, which may help the heart beat normally again.

If this doesn't help, or if the baby is not doing well and is big enough to deliver (thirty weeks into pregnancy or later), delivery is often the best way of handling the problem. After birth, many babies with congenital heart block lead normal lives with no treatment, but some need pacemakers.

Here it must be emphasized that the overall outlook is good for babies born to mothers who have Sjögren's. A blood test during pregnancy can identify anti-Ro and anti-La antibodies, and women who test negative can rest assured they will not have a child with neonatal lupus. Those who test positive for only the anti-Ro antibody should be aware of the possibility of rash and blood-test abnormalities in the child, but they should not worry unduly. For pregnant woman with both anti-Ro and anti-La antibodies, regular scans between weeks fifteen and twenty-five of pregnancy can check the baby's heartbeat (fetal echocardiography), and if an abnormality is detected, treatment by a specialist can be arranged as soon as possible for the best outcome.

Karen

After two miscarriages, I became and stayed pregnant. I was delighted, until during a routine scan during my twenty-eighth week the doctor was unable to find the baby's heartbeat. A scan and a fetal echocardiogram discovered that the baby had a heart block, although his heart had appeared and did still appear normal. I immediately had a blood test that showed I had Sjögren's syndrome—the first time I'd ever heard of it. The doctors explained that certain blood markers in my system were able to pass over into my baby's body and so affect his heart. I was taken into hospital until week thirty-four, when I had a caesarean to deliver the baby—some of the most anxious and depressing weeks of my life. Luckily he was fine and continues to be healthy and fit, with no need for a pacemaker or any other type of treatment.

After the Birth and Flare-Ups

In some cases, Sjögren's may flare after a birth, so it's a good idea to plan for this just in case. Have a look at the action plan for flare-ups in Chapter 6.

Your postpartum follow-up plan should include the following:

◆ Seeing your family doctor regularly and making any appointments you need with specialists

◆ Resuming exercise with the advice of your doctor

◆ Discussing with your doctor which medications, if any, you should be taking and if you can breast-feed your baby while taking them

◆ Knowing how much activity you can handle and how you can pace yourself to avoid exhaustion and stress

Adjusting to Motherhood

Patricia, mother of two

Those first few weeks after delivery were nothing like I'd imagined them to be. I thought I'd be able to get all the rest I needed because the baby would be so tiny and that the Sjögren's would take care of itself. Lack of sleep was the worst factor. It made me feel fluey and achy all the time. With my first baby, it took nearly six months for me to begin to adjust to my new life.

The combination of Sjögren's, loss of sleep, and the sheer impact of having a new person to care for can be exhausting. Don't expect too much of yourself and be sure to give yourself time to adapt to becoming a mother. Remember, mothers without Sjögren's suffer exhaustion and depression, too, but you may need to take extra care.

Taking Care of Yourself

◆ *Rest as much as you can.* If possible, take a nap when your child does. If you need to rest while your baby is awake, ask family, friends, or a hired person to care for her.

- *Get help during the first two weeks at the very least, and for a longer period of time if you can.* Another pair of hands is invaluable when washing up or for holding the baby while you shower. Get help from family and friends and make sure they understand your condition. Encourage any older children to get involved and to help. Think about employing somebody—maybe just a local teenager—to help you with the physical tasks involved in child care.

- *Leave the housework.* Yes, the house will need cleaning, and you'll wonder how such a small being can generate so much laundry, but it can be put off. A nap can be much more beneficial than sorting out the whites from the colors.

- *Put yourself first.* Make looking after yourself a priority. Let others take the baby for an hour while you relax in a warm bath or shower, get some sleep, have a nutritious meal or snack, or just spend some quiet time alone to recharge your battery.

- *Keep in touch.* Try to make time for old friends, even if it just involves a chat on the phone or an e-mail, and try to make new ones. Internet-based motherhood support groups are good, but real faces are even better. Look for local mother and baby groups or try and keep up with people you may have met at ante-natal classes.

Postpartum Depression

No one is quite sure what causes postpartum depression. Some blame hormones, others the psychological and social upheaval of becoming a mother. But while having a new baby should represent one of the happiest times of your life, it's true that some women—an estimated 10–20 percent—feel extra vulnerable, sad, or anxious after a birth. The enormous responsibility of a new baby to care for, combined with the strain of having a chronic condition and the sheer tiredness that can be involved, may be implicated. Family factors are also important, including your relationship with your partner and the level of support you may have from others.

On the third or fourth day after the baby is born, it's common to experience the baby blues—feeling weepy, sad, or irritable for no apparent reason. This often coincides with the arrival of your milk, and you may also run a slight temperature. Symptoms usually pass in a day or two.

It is important to distinguish the baby blues from postpartum depression, symptoms of which include the following:

◆ Feeling miserable, sad and tearful, that life is not worth living and you have nothing to look forward to

◆ Feeling that you can't cope

◆ Feeling guilty and irritable; snapping at your partner or other children

◆ Being constantly exhausted, often with disturbed sleep, including early morning waking

◆ Worrying about the baby and/or your own health

◆ Being unable to concentrate on anything or having a poor memory

◆ Feeling that your baby is a stranger and not really yours

◆ Having no interest in sex

◆ Finding it difficult to make decisions

◆ Having no appetite or engaging in comfort eating

If this is you, get help. Go to your family doctor or talk to your health visitor. Postpartum depression is treatable by medication, counseling, or both. The sooner treatment starts, the better things will be for you and your baby.

Baby Care

Aim to organize tasks so you expend the minimum amount of energy and effort. For example, you may find it difficult or painful to bend down and pick up the baby, or you may have a fear of dropping her. With time, you will find the baby-care methods that work best for you. It takes time to learn how to bathe, feed, and dress a new baby—all part of the process of becoming a mother, whether you have Sjögren's or not.

Bathing

Place the baby bath so it's level with you (i.e., on a worktop or in the sink), so you don't have to lean over, kneel, or reach up to bathe your baby. If the baby bath is in or near the sink, use a short hose or shower attachment to fill it. A wash mitt may help you wash your baby if you have hand problems. Wear an apron with large pockets to hold shampoo, soap, and other items. Sit on a high stool next to the sink while bathing the baby. If your baby just needs a sponge bath, put her in a car seat or bouncing chair.

Feeding

Use a pillow on your lap to support and raise your baby to make feeding easier. A chair with armrests will support your arms while holding him. You may find it easier to breast-feed lying on your side, rather than sitting upright and holding the baby.

If your feet are stiff and you find it hard to get out of bed for night feedings, do gentle range-of-motion exercises, especially to your ankles, before rising at night (see Chapter 8 for more on exercise). Keep a comfortable pair of slippers next to your bed. Ask your partner to bring the baby to you or ask him to handle the night-time feedings with a bottle of expressed breastmilk or formula. If you have hand problems, ask a family member to prepare a few baby bottles of breastmilk or formula in advance and keep the bottles in the refrigerator for the day.

Lifting and Carrying

If you suffer from joint pain and stiffness, lift and hold the baby with the arms rather than the hands to lessen the strain on the wrists and fingers. You may find it more comfortable to hold the baby close to you with both arms rather than with one.

Use a lightweight stroller that is easy to push and not so low that you have to bend down far to put your baby into it. A crib with low sides will make for easier picking up and laying down. If you raise the cot crib by placing it on a solid wood dais or something of similar construction, ensure the legs are firmly supported or secured so the crib can't wobble or move.

Don't put anything—baby included!—on the floor. If you place the baby on a waist-level surface, such as a bed, stay close by and surround her with pillows to prevent accidents. Your baby may learn to roll by three months and can take you by surprise!

Other Tips

- Use a wheeled cart or something similar to help you move equipment around the house.

- A front-worn sling may be better than holding the baby all the time. For you, it can mean more comfort, better posture, and a decreased likelihood of accidents. For your baby, it means closer contact and probably much less crying!

- Use room intercoms so you can hear your baby when he is sleeping. This will save you from walking to the baby's room every five minutes to check that he is all right.

- Keep items you need during the day for the baby, such as diapers and changes of clothes, in the area of your home where you will be most of the time, such as the kitchen.

- Babies grow quickly. Think ahead about baby-proofing

your home by, for example, covering electric sockets and fitting cupboards with locks.

◆ Discuss any problems with your doctor to see if they can help you find solutions.

Conclusion

The Future

Sjögren's syndrome is the second most common form of autoimmune disease after rheumatoid arthritis. Why do these bewildering diseases occur, and what can be done to reverse or halt them?

Research has a long way to go before finding answers. The root causes of autoimmune diseases are likely to be combinations of factors, both genetic and environmental. About 75 percent of autoimmune diseases are found in women, and women are more likely to get one autoimmune disease if they have a family member has also suffered from one. For example, your mother may have had lupus, while you have Sjögren's. A genetic predisposition to such diseases seems evident, but it is not that strong—the vast majority of people who have a relative with an autoimmune disorder will remain free of disease.

Other factors need to be taken into account in research. Some autoimmune diseases are known to begin or worsen with certain triggers, such as viral infections or the ingestion of certain medications. The severity or pattern of an autoimmune disease may be influenced by the genes a person inherits. It is thought that hormones play a role in inducing autoimmune diseases. Some cases, for instance, suddenly improve during pregnancy. Sometimes flare-ups occur after delivery, and other times a woman's Sjögren's will get worse during pregnancy or flare up after menopause. Other less-understood influences affecting the immune system and the course of autoimmune diseases include aging and stress. All of these offer areas for future research in order to increase our understanding of autoimmune diseases.

Research into Sjögren's is being pursued in many ways. Some workers are trying to unravel the genetic factors, while others are studying potential environmental triggers. Treatment research has focused on three main areas: first, to improve the efficacy and tolerability of artificial lubricants; second, to promote the secretion of the body's own tears and saliva; and third, to dampen down the body's immune and inflammatory responses.

Medical advances sometimes come from surprising sources—one of the most commonly used treatments for osteoporosis came from research into washing powders!—so who knows where the next breakthrough will come from?

But while scientific studies are ongoing, the most important researcher right now is you. By taking an active role in your treatment, noting your specific symptoms and finding out how best to deal with them, and exploring therapies and lifestyles that may help, you are well on the way to empowerment. And empowerment lies at the heart of healing.

Suggested Reading

Dauphin, Sue. *Understanding Sjögren's Syndrome*. Tequesta, FL: Pixel Press, 1993.

Fremes, Ruth, Nancy Carteron, and Arthur Grayzel. *A Body Out of Balance: Understanding and Treating Sjögren's Syndrome*. New York: Avery Publishing Group, 2003.

The Official Patient's Sourcebook on Sjögren's Syndrome: A Revised and Updated Directory for the Internet Age. San Diego, CA: Icon Health Publications, 2002.

Rumpf, Teri, and Kathy Hammit. *The Sjögren's Syndrome Survival Guide*. Oakland, CA: New Harbinger Publications, 2003.

Wallace, Daniel. *The New Sjögren's Syndrome Handbook*, 3rd ed. New York: Oxford University Press, 1998.

Resources

Organizations

American College of Rheumatology
1800 Century Pl., Suite 250
Atlanta GA 30345
(404) 633-3777
(404) 633-1870, fax
E-mail: acr@rheumatology.org
Website: www.rheumatology.org

National Family Caregivers Association (NCFA)
10400 Connecticut Ave., Suite 500
Kensington MD 20895
(800) 896-3650
(301) 942-6430
(301) 942-2302, fax
E-mail: info@thefamilycaregiver.org
Website: www.thefamilycaregiver.org

The National Institute of Arthritis and Musculoskeletal and Skin Diseases (NIAMS)
NIAMS/National Institutes of Health
1 AMS Circle
Bethesda MD 20892-3675
Website: www.niams.nih.gov

National Institutes of Health
Sjögren's Syndrome Clinic
10 Center Dr., MSC 1190
Building 10, Room 1N113
Bethesda MD 20892-1190
(301) 435-8528
Website: www.ninds.nih.gov

Sjögren's Syndrome Foundation
8120 Woodmont Ave., Suite 530
Bethesda MD 20814-1437
(301) 718-0300
(301) 718-0322, fax
E-mail: ssf@sjogrens.org
Website: www.sjogrens.org

Websites

Tips on Internet Searching

While the Internet is a source of useful information, you need to be discriminating and to read some pages with reservations. Some useful tips: The boxes at the side of the page are usually paid for, so the sites they bring you to may have a specific focus or even a product to push. The suffix .org implies a charity or an organization whose primary focus is not commercial. The suffix .ac or .edu implies an academic or educational site, likely to be well informed, but possibly narrow or esoteric in focus. Perhaps the most useful function of the Internet is its ability to put you in touch with others who live with Sjögren's.

Almark's page
Website: www.almark.net/sjogrens_syndrome_home.htm
This site features information on symptoms and diagnosis, some articles about the condition, links to other sites, and answers to frequently asked questions.

American Autoimmune Related Diseases Association (AARDA)
Website: www.aarda.org
The AARDA is the only national organization dedicated to the eradication of autoimmune diseases. AARDA sponsors physician's conferences, research, legislative advocacy, and a national awareness campaign to bring a national focus to autoimmunity.

The American College of Rheumatology
Website: www.rheumatology.org/directory/geo.asp
This site has an up-to-date regional listing of all members, enabling you to locate a rheumatologist in your area.

American Psychological Association Referral Service (APA)
Website: www.apa.org/practice/refer.html
Provides contact information for all state psychological associations, many of which have their own referral services.

Fibromyalgia (FM) Information from Oregon Fibromyalgia Foundation
Website: www.myalgia.com/sjogrens.htm
Information on FM and Sjögren's, including treatments.

Share
Website: www.NationalSHAREOffice.com
Supports those affected by early pregnancy loss, stillbirth, or newborn death.

Lynne's Sjögren's Syndrome
Website: http://lynne-sjogrens.org
A personal web page where people share their experiences of Sjögren's. Also includes information about symptoms, useful links, and helpful products.

Sjögren's Syndrome Foundation (SSF)
Website: www.sjogrens.org/support/
SSF sponsors over 100 support groups run by volunteers throughout the United States and Canada. The Foundation also has local volunteers who can provide information, education, and support by telephone.

Sjögren's World
Website: www.sjogrensworld.org
SjS World focuses primarily on the neurological manifestations of Sjögren's. The site offers articles and links, as well as E-Pals, discussion forums, instant messaging, live chats, and e-mail lists.

WebMD
Website: http://my.webmd.com/find_a_phys/doctor
This site enables you to search for a physician by specialty and region.

Index

Printed in the USA
CPSIA information can be obtained
at www.ICGtesting.com
JSHW082220140824
68134JS00015B/637